# The Missing Piece

# The Missing Piece

A Collection of Kidney Transplant Stories

Edited by Megan Podschlne

Cover by Kevin Woodland
Health Information Technology & Services
Michigan Medicine

Cover photo: Department of Communications
Michigan Medicine

Book design by Nicole Jacob
Health Information Technology & Services
Michigan Medicine

Produced by Health Information Technology & Services
Michigan Medicine

Published by Michigan Publishing
University of Michigan Library

ISBN 978-1-60785-390-9 (print)
ISBN 978-1-60785-485-2 (electronic)

# Dedication

This book is dedicated to Rob Rousseau and Celeste Lee.

Rob was a Patient Services Associate at the University of Michigan Transplant Center who put his heart and soul into his work. He was a great patient advocate whose mission was to make it easier for patients to receive the care they needed. His sense of humor and dedication to the job are irreplaceable. He has been greatly missed.

Celeste was a dedicated member of the Patient & Family Centered Care (PFCC) department. As the Program Manager for PFCC at Michigan Medicine (MM) and a patient with chronic kidney disease, she spent her life committed to making a difference for patients, families, and staff. She was a strong influence in helping with the kidney transplant peer mentor program. We greatly miss her knowledge and spirit.

# Contents

# Foreword

The miracle of kidney transplantation impacts people in many different ways. The recipient has renewed energy, a longer life expectancy, and is freed from the burdens—physical, emotional, and financial—of having to be on dialysis. The people who care about the recipient are uplifted and, in some ways, freed from the adverse impacts of end-stage renal disease on their own lives. Living donors can experience great pride and increased self-esteem in literally giving a part of themselves to help another human being. Families of deceased donors find the meaning and comfort that organ donation can bring in the face of a tragic event.

The joys and successes of transplant experiences are made even more compelling by the complexities of transplantation that make the journey more terrifying. The recipient must deal with anxiety that he or she may not be a candidate, that the transplant may fail, that a person may want to donate but cannot, or that someone may want to donate but is afraid of the risks. Recipients must face the possibility of not receiving a transplant and the reality that not all transplants last forever. There are complications, medication side effects, and other challenges that may occur.

As a transplant surgeon, I have had the privilege of seeing the impact of transplant firsthand. I have seen it in the physical appearance of the recipient, the satisfaction and pride of the living donor, and the joy of friends and families. We strive as medical professionals to make our work as routine as possible through precision, repetition, and experience, so that there is nothing that we can't handle. Yet, I am constantly reminded by the words and actions of transplant recipients and their families how much a kidney transplant is a life-changing event. The emotions can be overwhelming for all, even those of us who have experienced them over and over. Kidney transplantation remains one of the great thrills of my life.

The stories you will read here capture the breadth and depth of the transplant experience from a variety of perspectives. I have no doubt that, regardless of your background, you will be captivated, moved, and inspired by them. They serve as a great reminder to those of us in the transplant community that, despite all of the scientific, medical and technical advances that have been achieved, transplantation is above all else a uniquely human endeavor. It has a special meaning for all who are fortunate enough to experience it, either as a patient, family member, donor, relative of a deceased donor, or provider.

**Randall S. Sung, M.D.**
**Surgical Director of the Kidney Transplant Program**
**U-M Transplant Center**
**Michigan Medicine**

# Preface

In 2014, I was offered a position as Outreach Assistant at the University of Michigan (U-M) Transplant Center. At that time, I knew very little about the world of transplantation besides limited knowledge of a family member receiving a kidney from his sister. I was unfamiliar with the dire organ shortage and the small steps individuals can take to help save someone else's life.

Just a few years later, I am now working as a Project Manager at the U-M Transplant Center. I serve as the Program Manager of Wolverines for Life, a partnership between the University of Michigan community, Gift of Life Michigan, Eversight, the American Red Cross, Be the Match, and Team Michigan of the Donate Life Transplant Games of America to advocate for organ, tissue, blood, and bone marrow donation. I have organized several donor drives and have made it my mission to dispel the rumors and fears about donation.

During my time at the U-M Transplant Center, I have worked with referring physicians across the state to educate and inform them on the standard practices of transplantation as well as the latest advancements and technologies. I have worked with the community, student organizations, the public, and partner organizations to foster and grow the Michigan Organ Donor Registry. However, there is nothing more reassuring than to hear a patient speak about their experience after receiving a transplant. Patients are able to provide insight into the best and worst of their experiences, what we can do to improve, and how we can succeed together.

Working in this organization has allowed me to hear countless stories from kidney donors, recipients who received kidneys from living or deceased donors, and the family members of deceased persons who donated their organs. Although these stories are often bittersweet, it leaves me with a sense of purpose that even the worst of situations is an opportunity to turn someone else's life around.

I encourage all of you to please join the Michigan Organ Donor Registry at www.giftoflifemichigan.org/go/umhs. If you do not have a Michigan Identification Card or Driver's License, please visit registerme.org to join Donate Life's national organ donor registry.

**Megan Podschlne**
**Project Manager**
**U-M Transplant Center**
**Michigan Medicine**

# Acknowledgements

Thank you to the University of Michigan (U-M) Transplant Center Kidney Team for their contributions and support of this book. The authors of these stories are able to tell their stories thanks to your care and compassion. Thank you to Dr. Randall Sung, the Surgical Director of the Kidney Transplant Program, for writing the Foreword to this book and sharing your wisdom and experience with us all.

Thank you to Bob Garypie for taking the team photo following this Acknowledgement. I appreciate your willingness to find time to help out with this project and to make it fun for everyone involved, even if it's just making a goofy face while facing a wall.

I would especially like to thank Stacy Brand, Outreach Manager of the U-M Transplant Center; Colleen Satarino, kidney transplant Social Worker; and the pre-transplant coordinators and living donor coordinators for their help in finding patient authors of varying backgrounds. A special thank you to Stacy for being a second set of eyes through the editing process.

I would also like to thank Jasna Markovac, formerly of Michigan Medicine, now at California Institute for Technology, for approaching us with this idea. Jasna got the ball rolling with this project and made it clear how we could help ease the fears and anxieties of those considering transplant.

I am very grateful for the Publishing Editors of the Documentation and Publishing department of HITS at Michigan Medicine. Their patience and understanding, as we slowly crawled through the process of compiling this book, were astounding. They were always available to answer my questions, even when I didn't know I had them.

Finally, I would like to thank our authors for sharing their stories and reliving their experiences. I hope they were able to look back and be proud of their accomplishments and how far they have come. I am so glad I was able to work on this project with each of you and hear about such an important period of your life.

**Megan Podschlne**

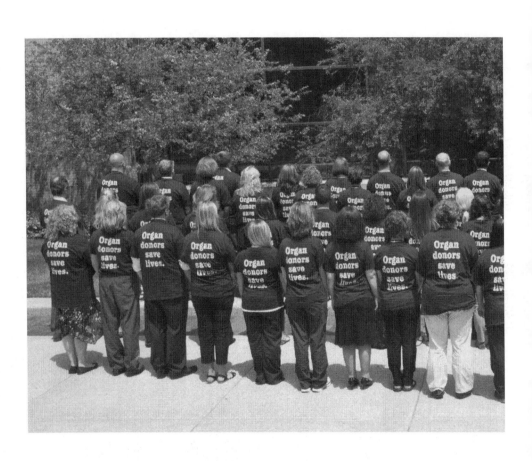

University of Michigan Transplant Center staff and faculty gathering to celebrate organ donation and transplantation.

Photo Credit: Bob Garypie, University of Michigan Transplant Center

## Kidney Waitlist vs. Transplants

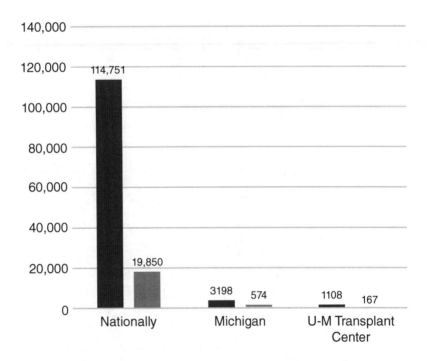

Number of people on waitlist (as of 5/18/18)
Number of people transplanted (throughout 2017)

Source: United Network for Organ Sharing

# Introduction

In 1964, Janice Ottenbacher received a kidney from her identical twin sister, Joan Ottenbacher, as the University of Michigan's first kidney transplant surgery. At the time, this was a cutting-edge procedure, only ten years after the first kidney transplant surgery in history took place in Boston, Massachusetts. More than fifty years after the surgery, both women are thriving. They both went on to become nurses and create their own families.

Since then, we have made many advancements in transplant surgery. Transplant centers around the world are now performing transplant surgeries on nonrelated donors by tissue typing organs. They have established paired donation programs for nonmatching donors and recipients, and they continue to make improvements to medicinal aftercare.

The Paired Donation Program allows multiple, unmatched donor-and-recipient pairs to donate to others. For example, Donor A would like to donate a kidney to Recipient A but is not a match. Donor B would like to donate a kidney to Recipient B but is also not a match. If Donor A matches Recipient B and Donor B matches Recipient A, the system identifies them and both pairs have the opportunity to donate to one another. The transplant surgeries are coordinated so all parties donate or receive a kidney at the same time. The Paired Donation chain can continue to grow when more matches are made and altruistic donors become involved. According to ScienceDaily, the longest paired donation chain contained thirty donors and thirty recipients in a nationwide exchange.

However, there is still a considerable amount of work to be done. A disproportionate number of people are being added to the national transplant waiting list compared to those receiving transplants. According to the United Network for Organ Sharing, someone is added to the national transplant waiting list every ten minutes; an average of twenty people die each day waiting for a transplant.

Through research and development, we are making strides to conquer the current organ shortage, but we still must focus on the patients waiting for a transplant today. By joining the organ donor registry, you have the opportunity to save up to eight lives. If you are interested in joining the organ donor registry, please visit the Michigan registry:
giftoflifemichigan.org/go/umhs
Or visit the national registry:
registerme.org

Almost all major religions support organ donation or leave it to the discretion of the individual and/or the individual's family. For more information about religious viewpoints on organ donation, visit:
unos.org/donation/facts/theological-perspective-on-organ-and-tissue-donation/

We encourage those needing a kidney transplant to discuss the possibility of a living donation with their friends and family. This is one way we can expedite the process of receiving a transplant. There are many benefits to living donations, including a longer lifespan for the transplanted kidney, more flexibility in scheduling the surgery, and a shorter amount of time spent on dialysis. There are minimal risks associated with the donor surgery. We encourage you to call the U-M Transplant Center if you are interested in finding out if you may be a potential donor. For the donor, the University of Michigan (U-M)

# Introduction

Transplant Center will cover all expenses related to the kidney donation and any subsequent complications.

Since Joan and Janice's transplant in 1964, the U-M Transplant Center has performed over 6,600 kidney transplant surgeries, even working abroad to develop a kidney transplant clinic in Ethiopia. In 2015, a team of physicians and nurses flew from the U-M Transplant Center to perform the first kidney transplant in Ethiopia at St. Paul's Hospital Millennium Medical College in Addis Ababa. St. Paul's staff worked for two years to develop the transplant clinic and train local medical professionals.

Michigan Medicine has one of the oldest and largest transplant programs in the country. We have performed over 11,000 transplants including heart, lung, liver, kidney, pancreas, and cornea and recently introduced a hand transplant program.

Whether you are a patient waiting for a kidney transplant, a caregiver helping someone through this process, or a concerned friend, I hope you enjoy reading these patient stories from a small group of our patients about their lives before and after their transplant surgeries. These individuals come from various backgrounds, each with their own experiences and aspirations. *Those with chronic kidney disease did not let it stop them from living their lives.* Instead, they faced this adversity with the willpower to move past it. They used their resources—sometimes hesitantly—to improve their situations and their quality of life. These are not just patients, donors, and recipients. They are heroes.

**Megan Podschlne**

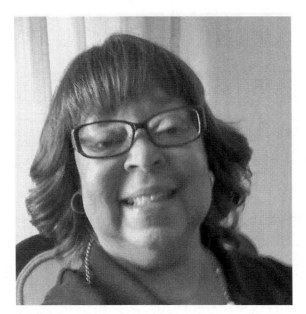

Armethyst

# Armethyst's Story

Armethyst was diagnosed with lupus nephritis and received a transplant at 57 years old from a deceased donor.

My journey began in the mid-1990s, when I was functioning on autopilot taking care of my daughter, mother, grandmother, and critically ill husband. Like many other people, I felt the stress of keeping a full-time job and trying to meet all my other responsibilities. When I began feeling fatigued, I went to the doctor expecting a shot or some vitamins. To my surprise I was diagnosed with chronic fatigue syndrome (CFS). Later it was changed to systemic lupus, an autoimmune disease that attacks healthy organs.

Initially, my fatigue was the only presenting symptom so I compartmentalized the situation and felt as if this was going to be my new normal. I was not fully aware of how lupus would impact my life until I had my first flare. It was an eye-opening experience. It felt like a bomb exploded and every joint in my body was inflamed. I now had debilitating fatigue. The fatigue was so intense that I could no longer take care of anyone else. I could barely take care of myself.

I struggled with everyday tasks. Just to make it from my car to my office was a Herculean feat. I was put on a new regimen of medications to help stabilize the lupus. I remember feeling that sometimes the side effects of the medications were more difficult than the disease itself. I began to feel anxious regarding my future independence. I forced myself to stay in the present and not let my mind wander.

After about six years of trying to manage my lupus, I began to have symptoms of kidney failure, and I sought the help of a nephrologist. My family tried to be supportive, but it was difficult for them to understand what I was experiencing with lupus. I did not want my daughter in the role of being my caretaker or worrying about me, so I encouraged her to go to college out of state.

When I began working with a nephrologist, I was taught to read my lab reports so I could understand the progress of my kidney disease. I was placed on a kidney diet, which let me feel like I was prolonging my time before needing dialysis.

When it was time for me to begin to dialyze, I was given a choice between hemodialysis or peritoneal dialysis. I chose peritoneal dialysis because I could do it in the comfort of my home without assistance. This process had no blood, pain, or needles. It involved manually exchanging fluids through my stomach four times a day, seven days a week.

I was even able to dialyze at work during my lunch hour. During this period, I experienced unexpected compassion and support from my coworkers. They were encouraged by my dear friend and coworker, Ruthann. She provided constant support and counsel and was there any time I was hospitalized. My daughter, now a young lady, was my rock. Her support kept me going.

The deciding factor for me to pursue placement on the transplant list was that I wanted to live a better quality of life and a longer life. I recognized that the average stay on the list was five years, but I was willing to try. The University of Michigan Transplant Center began testing to qualify me for the list. This involved completing a number of tests that examined every inch of my body to ensure I would be safe if

I had a transplant. I had several chronic health issues, but I still qualified for an alternative kidney, one that was no longer pristine. I was satisfied with whatever option I was offered. The University of Michigan Health System (UMHS) staff were wonderful about answering questions and helping me through the process. So, I was placed on the organ transplant waitlist.

I remember sitting at my office desk on December 26, 2007, and getting a telephone call from the county sheriff informing me that UMHS was looking for me. I had a kidney waiting. I cannot even express to you my emotions. It was overwhelming. When I got to the hospital, they prepared me and whisked me off for surgery. Luckily, I was able to see my daughter and my friend, Ruthann, just before I was given anesthesia.

The recovery went well. I was walking the hospital halls the next day. The hospital staff used this time to educate me about my wonderful gift, my responsibilities, and my limitations. I had received my kidney from a 64-year-old gentleman who was deceased. His family graciously allowed me to have this gift of life. I am forever grateful and give thanks to them daily for such a precious gift.

After I received my kidney transplant, I immediately felt more energetic than I had in years. I could walk without losing my breath, and the brain fog was lifted. People commented that my skin coloring was different.

This is my tenth year after getting my kidney. Once you receive your transplant, you need to be diligent in taking your antirejection medications. You also should be mindful of your suppressed immune system. Transplanted individuals are medically monitored for the rest of their lives. Monthly lab tests are required to determine if the medication levels are balanced and to assess the function of the transplant.

Rejection is always a possibility. I won't say that it was all smooth sailing, but I never regretted my decision.

It is important to remember that no major religion objects to transplantation. It is also important to remember that if one has an illness, this doesn't necessarily prohibit you from donating an organ, tissue, or other parts of the body.

My journey is not complete. I look forward to many more years, hopefully with this kidney. I want to thank the University of Michigan Transplant Center for their care and support. They continue to ensure that I am able to realize my goal of a better quality of life.

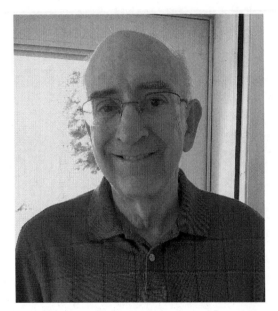

Bob

# Bob's Story

Bob was diagnosed with type 2 diabetes and hypertensive nephrosclerosis. He received a transplant at 63 years old from an altruistic living donor.

I had my kidney transplant on October 15, 2014. It went very well and I have recovered very nicely. It all began approximately two and a half years before my transplant. I am not exactly sure what brought it to my doctor's attention—I think it was my high creatinine level (a measure of kidney function) that started the whole thing. I remember my primary care doctor meeting me in the recovery room at the hospital and telling me he was going to have me evaluated to be put on the waiting list.

"What list?" I asked.

He said, "The kidney transplant list."

When I asked why, he stated it was as a precaution.

My awareness of my right-side kidney problems began a few months before that. I am a typical doctor who does not take care of himself. My kidneys were failing because of my diabetes. I really did not take the waitlist situation seriously but I went through the procedures, as requested, and was evaluated by the University of Michigan (U-M) Transplant Center.

My two sons volunteered to be donors. Neither of them turned out to be a match. I continued life as normal, and I started seeing a nephrologist who monitored my condition. Although my creatinine continued to rise, my heart function stayed normal, and I was able to avoid dialysis. I continued my daily work schedule as normal.

At the end of August 2014, my nephrologist advised me to go on dialysis. I asked him to give me one more month, and he agreed. I was going to use the peritoneal method because, as a surgeon, I did not want them using the vessels in my arms.

On September 15, 2014, I decided he was right and I could not go on like this because I was just too tired. I needed dialysis. The very next day I got a call from U-M Transplant Center telling me they had a perfect donor for me. Since it was a living donor, we could immediately plan the next step.

I had met my transplant surgeon weeks before the surgery. He was very personable and very well trained, as would be expected, and very smart.

The donor was a 27-year-old female who was working at a hospital that had quite a few dialysis patients. She decided to donate a kidney, and I was a match. I was on the list for approximately two and a half years before this event. I spent the next month finishing up the work I needed to complete before taking time off from work.

I showed up at the appointed time for my surgery, which took place around 4:00 p.m. I remember nothing from the point when they said, "We're ready for you," until the next day when I woke up in my room with my wife next to me. I was told the surgery took two hours. I was feeling great. For the first time, I realized how sick I really was. My creatinine was coming back to normal.

I was in the hospital until Saturday morning. My post-op care was excellent. I had no pain and didn't need to take pain medication.

My recovery at home was completely uneventful. I had a great private-duty nurse—my wife—who took excellent care of me. I was assigned a transplant nephrologist at U-M Transplant Center. Her team took excellent care of me. They were always accessible to my needs and my post-op visits were uneventful. Postoperatively, my kidney function was perfect. My only problems have been related to my compromised immune system, which leaves me vulnerable to viruses.

I will never have a direct comparison because I do not plan to have this done again. But I can say in all honesty, as a doctor in surgery, I cannot imagine anyone doing it better than the U-M Transplant Center. They have a saying at the university, "It's the team, the team, the team." Of course, they were talking about football, but they should have been talking about the kidney transplant team.

I am back to working full-time. I went back to work on December 1, 2014. I hope this little story will help anybody else going down this road.

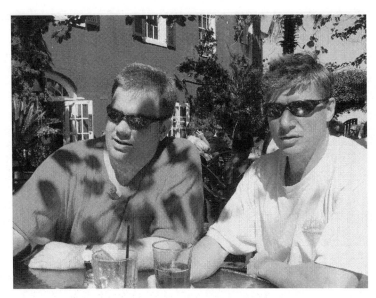

Carsten (left) and Bernhard (right)

# Carsten's Story

Carsten was diagnosed with hydronephrosis and received his first transplant at 26 years old and a second at 46 years old. Both transplants were from living donors.

"You're still a young woman. You can have other children. This one is not going to make it."

I'm paraphrasing, but this is what my mother heard after taking me to the pediatrician when I was nine months old. The situation was grave—it was discovered that I had only one kidney and a ureter blockage was destroying it. An emergency surgery was able to get urine flowing again, but the damage to the kidney was extensive. What followed over the next few years were several more surgeries to keep the kidney functioning. I hit my teens and the kidney seemed to be holding its own. Then, at college, I contracted mononucleosis, and the kidney began to fail. Through extensive dietary restrictions I was able to keep it going for another seven years, at which point it was time to consider transplantation. That was 1991. Although my brother was a good match, the decision was made to use my mother's kidney since she was still young enough to donate, and I would likely need another kidney before "my time."

I was 26 when the transplant took place. In retrospect, I think I took it fairly lightly (at 26 I was still immortal, after all). My mother worried enough for the both of us, and I used my sense of humor to keep the situation light. One memory I have is when she and I were at University of Michigan Health System (UMHS) for orientation day. While waiting in line at the blood-drawing station and looking through the paperwork,

I commented: "Wow, mom, they give a free, round-trip ticket on Delta with every transplant!" The woman in front of us turned around and asked in amazement, "Really??" We must have laughed for a good ten minutes.

When you have a chronic condition that affects your health over years and years, it's hard to notice how bad things have gotten. That was the case for me. I was amazed with how much energy and vitality I felt after the transplant. The removal of all the dietary restrictions was wonderful, too, and I can still taste that first bite of a fast-food cheeseburger after not having been able to enjoy them for the better part of a decade!

Fast-forward twenty years to 2011. The transplanted kidney had been doing great, it had been another fun summer of travel, and I was looking at the potential of an exciting new career with one of the auto makers. My creatinine had been up a tick for the past couple of months, but it was likely not a big deal. I was waiting for the biopsy results to prove it. Instead, I was told that, within roughly the next six months, the kidney from my mother was going to fail. The cause? Transplant glomerulopathy. I had never even heard of it, but apparently it is one of the major causes of transplant kidney failure. I was stunned.

Although my brother, Bernhard, was a prime candidate to donate, how does one go about asking his physically fit, marathon-running, airline-pilot sibling to go through his first major surgery on your behalf? Thankfully, my mother spilled the beans. My brother was furious that I had even remotely considered not asking him to donate.

"If the roles were reversed, would you give me a kidney?"

"Well, of course I would," I replied.

That settled it. We both breathed a sigh of relief when the bloodwork showed that he was still a great match twenty-one years after he was first tested. Again, we used sense of humor to offset the nervousness during the day-long orientation. As the nurse was addressing the room of patients and talking about the size of the donor's incision, my brother turned to me and stammered, "Incision? You never told me there would be an incision!"

Anesthesia. Surgery. Hospital. Transplant. These words have such an emotional impact because of the fact that we understand so little about the complexities of our bodies. Yet they are what give us life, which is why we are so protective of them.

As I write this summary of my transplant history I'm also watching a technician work on our office printer/copier/scanner, a behemoth of a machine that I barely know how to insert paper into. He is expertly flipping levers, popping out components, cleaning them, and replacing them, using a set of specialty tools and his knowledge and experience to guide him. It occurs to me that, as scary as those hours before surgery felt, I was in the hands of a team of people who also had specialty tools, knowledge, and experience, only this time for the machine known as "me." That surgeon who was about to perform a laparoscopic nephrectomy on my brother? He likely was going to perform that procedure as fluidly and efficiently as the technician who is working on our copier right now. The nursing staff that was going to receive us on floor 5C after recovery? Again, thanks to their knowledge and experience, our odds of full recovery and zero complications were high.

The surgery took place two weeks before Easter in 2012. As before, everything went flawlessly, and both my brother and I are doing fine five years later. Once again, the slow erosion of my physical health has vanished and although the immunosuppressive medications add complexities to my life I hadn't expected (significant precautions against skin cancer along with annual cancer screenings and visits to dermatology), the rewards of my UMHS kidney transplant far outweigh the risks.

Those rewards even extend to my relationship with my brother. We have developed a closeness that was missing from our relationship before. He lives in Phoenix now, but we see each other regularly and talk on the phone at least once a week. We commemorate the transplant every Thanksgiving by attending the Detroit Lions game together here in Detroit (they have won every year we have attended), followed by a meal with a family that I am truly thankful for. As it turns out, I got much more than just a kidney that Wednesday morning back in 2012.

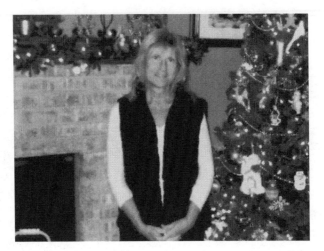

Eve

# Eve's Story

Eve was diagnosed with polycystic kidney disease and received a transplant at 57 years old from a deceased donor.

If I've learned anything in life, it's that no matter who you are—young or old, rich or poor—life will, at some point, throw at least one good punch at you. It is how you handle it that counts. I would say I have pretty much skimmed along quite easily in life, being blessed with loving parents, a wonderful husband, and two beautiful daughters who I managed to stay at home with while watching them grow into two beautiful young women. No health problems, no personal problems, a steady job. Yes, life was on a very even keel, until a routine physical exam in 2004 led to a routine abdominal ultrasound just to check out a little bit of hardness in my liver area. I was a bit puzzled when the technician asked if I knew of any kidney problems in my family history. I answered, "No," and didn't think any more of it.

A couple of days later my doctor called me and stated that I had polycystic kidney disease (PKD). This meant I would have to have more frequent check-ups and lab draws for monitoring purposes. It didn't sink in at all. I had no knowledge of this disease and, quite frankly, didn't receive any further information about it at first. I happened to mention it to my family, but we never grasped the seriousness or final outcome of what having kidney disease meant for my future. I was instructed to watch my diet and was given blood pressure medication since my blood pressure was always on the high side, even in my youth.

The doctor's call got me thinking. Polycystic kidney disease is a genetic disease. So, who in my family had a history of kidney disease? I mentally ticked off any health problems on both sides of my family. A little nagging feeling started to bother me as I thought about my father's health issues during his lifetime: high blood pressure, water retention, kidney stones, diverticulosis, and most importantly, dying from kidney failure after a non–life-threatening surgery. He never mentioned having any kidney problems to me, but it finally started sinking in that I may be in trouble.

When I was finally referred to a nephrologist, she filled me in on the seriousness of this disease and the potentially life-threatening prognosis that lay ahead. In other ways, I was in good health and was advised to consider becoming a candidate for a kidney transplant. Otherwise, she said, I would eventually require dialysis at some point down the road. I needed to take action if I wanted to extend my years on this planet, not only for my sake, but also for my family's.

I got in touch with the University of Michigan (U-M) Transplant Center and joined a small group of individuals for a class regarding the transplant process. At this point, I was a bit smug, thinking I was with a group of people who I believed were obviously sicker than I was. Most of them were already on dialysis. I thought I would be put on the transplant list, but of course, that would be much later in the future. I think I will call this my "denial" stage, as I just could not or would not process all this information coming at me. Nevertheless, I went through all the testing required. I was considered healthy enough to make the list! The wait time? On average, I was told, about five years in Michigan.

With that taken care of, life went pretty smoothly for the next six years. Although, during that time, my lab results were getting closer to Stage 2, Stage 3, and in November of 2010, just days before celebrating becoming an American citizen, I was informed that my kidney disease had rapidly deteriorated to Stage 4. I was to start dialysis immediately. My head was spinning! Before I knew it, I had a catheter sticking out from beneath my neck, covered by an immensely bulging bandage— a constant reminder of the inevitable.

I quietly informed my boss that I would have to adjust my schedule so I could go to dialysis three times a week after work. This would take place every week during a 40-hour busy work week at a medical practice. My family was very supportive, but in shock. They, too, had to deal with the fact that this would affect their lives, not just mine. I wouldn't be available to tend to my family's needs or go to social events on dialysis days. And any vacations to farther destinations would have to include dialysis treatments. I would experience fatigue, nausea, vomiting, dizziness, excruciating muscle cramps, and those darn needles being stuck into me. But at least I was well enough to continue working full-time.

I had great support from my family, friends, and dialysis staff and a newfound positive attitude. No matter what, I would never take a single day for granted, and I continually counted my blessings. Most importantly, I never ever missed treatment! Being compliant was first and foremost in my plan to keep myself as healthy as possible throughout this journey until the day that I would receive "the call" from the U-M Transplant Center.

I finally did receive that wonderful phone call just five days before Christmas in 2014. Yes, be prepared for that life-changing phone call. It can happen at any moment, day or night. My husband had just stepped on the ice, ready to play hockey in his over-50 league when he received my news and had to anxiously drive back home to take me to the hospital. Everything happened so fast from then on. My transplant was a miraculous success. I did not receive only one kidney, but rather, two healthy kidneys from a little child. I thank God every day for her family's decision to save my life. My "twins," as I call them, began functioning immediately. I was out of the hospital and able to go home on Christmas Day. Not only could I be home to celebrate Christmas, but I could also be with my mother, who was visiting from Canada. She got to see, firsthand, the wonderful treatment I received from the entire U-M Transplant Center. While I was off work recovering, I also had the loving companionship of my beloved furry angel, Fiona, my dear kitty whose job it was to help in my healing process. She came to our family just a month before my transplant, thanks to my wise and loving husband, and has been my faithful companion ever since.

It's been just over two years since I received my kidney transplant, and I continue to feel rejuvenated and so grateful to get a second chance to live a full and happy life. As I have found out, life carries uncertainties, which we have to come to terms with, and I don't know how long my kidneys will continue functioning. I just take each day one at a time, continue being thankful, remain compliant in taking my immunosuppressants, get my monthly blood draws, and ask God each day to guide my steps to that certain person who needs a sympathetic ear, encouragement, a hug, or just a smile.

Yes, this has been a life-changing and humbling journey, one that I can truly say I am thankful for. I've since learned a few things I would like to share.

First, take control. It's totally up to you to manage your treatment and your attitude. Gaining as much knowledge as possible about your disease and subsequent treatment will ease your fears about the unknown. Deciding to have a positive attitude makes an enormous difference in how you feel, but don't think that you have to tackle this all by yourself. Be open to receiving the support you need from whatever sources make you feel comfortable.

Be open to giving of yourself, too. Reach out to those who need encouragement and empathy. You'll be surprised how good it makes you feel by being a blessing to others. You will be blessed in return. I guarantee it!

It is important to feel reassured that you have people rooting for you and willing to offer whatever help you will need along your journey.

Second, be compliant. I can't stress enough how important it is to follow your medical team's instructions. This means going to all your dialysis treatments and then taking your immunosuppressant medications as instructed every day after you receive your transplant. Take care of yourself! Modern medical science has given you the opportunity to defy what was, in the past, a certain and inevitable death sentence. You can prolong your life by many years with the treatment that is best for you.

Third, this is for all those who are healthy individuals: whether you decide to donate a kidney while you're alive or after death, you can be certain you have made a wonderful contribution to saving someone's life!

I am grateful to have the opportunity to share my kidney transplant journey and give thanks to the U-M Transplant Center and everyone involved with the transplant process, from beginning to end and beyond. I hope you know you are truly appreciated and always will be. Over the years there have been so many people I've known, and those I wasn't even aware of, who prayed for me and kept me close to their hearts. If it wasn't for my diagnosis, I would never have known how many cared about me and my well-being.

I am most grateful to my husband, daughters, my dear Mummy, extended family, and friends for their constant love, support, and encouragement throughout my experiences during these last 13 years since my diagnosis. I hope my story gives hope and encouragement to those of you who have been diagnosed with kidney disease and that it gives you the strength you need as you go through your own personal journey.

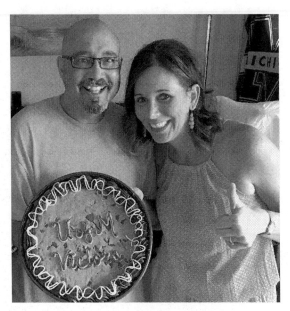

David (left) and Tricia (right)

# David's Story

David was diagnosed with IgA nephropathy (Berger's disease). He received a transplant at 28 years old from a living donor and at 43 years old from a living donor in the paired donor program.

My name is David. I am 45 years old and a two-time kidney transplant recipient. Let me tell you a little more about me and my journey to recovery. In 1997, at the young, wide-eyed age of 25, I was first diagnosed with chronic kidney failure. Severe migraines were mainly what led me to seek advice from medical experts. At that time, I was told it was serious, and I immediately started on full-time dialysis. It was overwhelming to get news this severe, as I had no idea what to expect when I first went to the hospital with my dad.

I was working full-time on the assembly line at an RV factory. I worked for as long as I could, but being on dialysis made it extremely difficult to maintain a regular work schedule. My kidneys were permanently damaged; therefore, my sudden diagnosis left me no choice but to seek a kidney transplant. At one point, doctors traced it back to a case of mononucleosis (mono) and strep throat when I was in my teens.

Once I wrapped my brain around things, my optimism quickly took over, and so began our search and placement on the kidney transplant registry. It did not take long for my mom to step up and offer hers. She was determined about it and further testing revealed she was also a good match. There was no arguing with my mother.

In early 2000, the transplant surgery was performed at University of Michigan Health System (UMHS) in Ann Arbor, Michigan. The operation was a complete success for us both. It was no shock to me seeing as I am a die-hard U of M fan.

Really, most people don't realize how debilitating kidney disease is. The transplant made all the difference in the world and, thanks to my mom, I was given a second chance at life. She and many others made good jokes reminding me of the sacrifice she made for me.

I soon returned to work. My daily routine included taking antirejection medicines and other drugs. For the most part, I felt like myself again, and I finally had my life back on track. When I first received the kidney from my mom, I was told all about the success rates and risks. I knew the kidney may not work forever but that wasn't something I thought about much during that time or dwelled on in my future plans.

Little did I know that by 2013 my transplanted kidney would fail. It did not take long for me to realize it had happened. I was not experiencing migraines like the first time around, but I did have severe swelling in my legs and knew something was wrong. At that time, "optimistic" is still the best word to describe how I felt at that moment. I suppose I could have felt shocked or disappointed, but after all, with the help of my mom, I had successfully handled one kidney transplant.

I began my search for a second chance at a normal life. I was once again placed on full dialysis and again had to step away from my full-time job to begin the full-time grind of dialysis. I had the support of many close friends, a devoted wife, and family. However, due to some new developments with my two brothers, finding a good match with another family member or friend did not seem very likely. We had found out that my kidney failure was possibly related to a genetic condition known as IgA Berger's disease. This made it very difficult for another family member to step forward. I had several acquaintances from work and my church offer to donate a kidney, but after the initial testing and evaluation process none made the cut.

In July of 2013, my family and friends hosted a benefit for me at a local church in my hometown. I reconnected with a high school acquaintance and, just like my mom, there was no arguing with her, either. I was on full dialysis for almost two years before I received my second transplant. Once the surgery was complete, I felt like a million bucks! This second transplant was part of a three-way paired donation that occurred between UMHS and two other local hospitals.

As I reflect on my journey and both of my roads to recovery, I am grateful for my health. I feel better than I have since I was 25 years old. I have a positive outlook despite a little fear that when the time comes for my next kidney my friends will be too old to donate. In the meantime, I am planning to return to work full-time and to pursue a new business venture. I travel often and am living a great life!

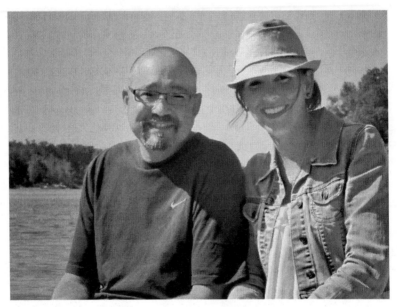

David (left) and Tricia (right)

# Tricia's Story

Tricia was 42 years old when she was a donor in the paired donation program with David.

My name is Tricia. I am 44 years old, a wife, and mother of three active teenage boys. It was July of 2013, and I had just returned to my hometown for our annual Fourth of July festivities at the lake. I heard they were having a benefit for a lifelong friend of mine, David. He and I met in the 8th grade and were close friends all through high school and the early college years. I am ashamed to say I had lost touch with him over the past few years so had truly no idea what he was up against.

I still clearly remember walking into the very crowded room, hugging him, and asking him what exactly was going on. He quickly caught me up to speed and simply stated he "was in need of a new kidney." Without a moment's hesitation I asked him if I could donate mine. Because of our blood types, we knew right away we couldn't do a direct exchange. He pulled a cocktail napkin from the buffet and proceeded to explain to me as simply as possible exactly how a paired donation could work. I tucked the napkin and drawing into my purse and headed to the food line, determined that I would do whatever it took to make this happen. He did not argue with me—we had been friends for way too long, and he knew better than that.

For me, the decision was simple—my friend needed help, and I could help him. Say no more. I called the University of Michigan Health

System (UMHS) on Monday and set up an appointment to be tested and evaluated. In all honesty, that was the easy part.

The difficult part was explaining to my husband and immediate family my desire to make this sacrifice. They, of course, were concerned for my own health and well-being. Reluctantly, my husband agreed to attend the initial testing and screening with me in September of 2013. I passed the tests and listened as they explained the process of how the kidney exchange program worked. Even though my kidney would not be directly received by David, there was an opportunity for this to benefit not only one person, but multiple!

I felt a complete sense of purpose to be a part of something so life-changing. At no point did I ever feel reluctant or think I would take it back. I felt confident in my own health, in the genetics of my family, and that neither I nor my three boys would be harmed in any way, now or in the future. I thought of David's mother—who was a mother of three boys, like me. I imagined how difficult and painful it must have been to be faced with this obstacle again. My decision was so simple, as I knew this would bring much joy to her as well. My husband and immediate family were still uncertain but remained very supportive through the process.

It was not until late Spring of 2015 that we received the call that a match had been found. The overall process did take longer than I had anticipated, but not once did I have a second thought. I had some repeat testing done during that time just to be sure my health had not changed drastically. I still had the green light and was physically and emotionally more than ready. My friend, David, at that time was doing dialysis on a full-time basis, and I could see it taking a toll on him.

Our surgeries were performed on July 22, 2015. We had the good fortune of being two of six in a three-way exchange with two other donors pairs who were, ironically, all in the same area. I truly had no idea what to expect. I was fortunate to have not had the experience of surgery and, other than three natural births of my boys, had never even been in a hospital before. The staff and doctors at UMHS were extremely kind and helpful and the surgeries involving all six of us were a monumental success.

My recovery was remarkably uneventful. My husband, family, and friends were very supportive and within a week I had returned to most of my normal duties with the exception of very strict weight limitations and other minor restrictions. David and I were both doing so well that we attended a service at his church only four days after our surgeries. His sense of humor was evident as he proceeded to tell the entire congregation how thankful he was to me for his "newfound ability to pee" once again.

Physically, I feel no different. I maintain a healthy diet, exercise often, and continue to drink lots of water. Emotionally, it is hard to put into words the extreme sense of satisfaction and fulfillment. I only wish I had another kidney to give. The highlight of the journey was meeting the other donors and recipients in October of 2015.

I would encourage anyone considering kidney donation to just do it. You will be glad you did.

Editor's Note: University of Michigan Health System and two other local hospitals collaborated to perform a three-way paired kidney donation. Three individuals needed a kidney and three individuals were willing to donate but weren't a match for their loved ones. Thanks to the paired kidney donation process, three transplants were able to take place within a few hours of each other.

# Fairy's Story

Fairy was diagnosed with type 2 diabetes and hypertensive nephrosclerosis. She received a transplant at 64 years old from a deceased donor.

I was devastated when I was told I had kidney problems. I was already dealing with diabetes. All kinds of questions were in my mind. I did not have any answers to the question, "Why?" I don't drink, and I don't smoke. I'm a firm believer that God doesn't put any more on you than you can bear. Sometimes things just happen, and only God knows the answer.

This is one of those times.

The doctor's diagnosis was that I had too much calcium in my blood and too much protein in my urine. My kidneys could not flush out the amount of fluids that were necessary to function properly. The calcium caused one of my parathyroid glands to enlarge due to overproduction of calcium. This process destroyed my kidney, and surgery was required to remove it.

For several years, controlling my diet helped to slow down the kidney disease process. Unfortunately, this was not enough to stop the deterioration of my kidney to the point that my doctor and I decided that I should go on dialysis.

I am a very strong person and did not want to burden my family. When they became aware of my condition, they were devastated. I became very depressed, confused, and disappointed. I was praying that I would not have to go on dialysis. One thing I know is that God doesn't give you any more than you can bear. So my question wasn't, "Why?" I don't question God. Whatever His will, "It shall be done."

After many days of meditation and prayer, I did my first hemodialysis treatment on July 5, 2005. I dialyzed on Tuesdays, Thursdays, and Fridays for three and a half hours a day. Dialysis days were not easy. They drained me of all my energy. It was as if I was a normal, functional person every other day.

Then I went on peritoneal dialysis nightly for more than six years. I did this treatment for myself, never asking for the assistance of family members. Sometimes I was confused and depressed, but through it all I relied on the Lord. I was never alone. I knew God was going to bring me through.

Storing more than thirty boxes of solution, tubing, and other supplies in my house for my dialysis treatment meant making one bedroom free for storage. These treatments were for 10–12 hours nightly, with one legal time off for thirty minutes.

*Ecc. 3:1 "To everything there is a season and a time to every purpose under the heaven."*

This was my season—my time.

During those years, I was able to continue functioning and doing the things I enjoyed daily. This gave me a little freedom. Although it was confining, it was what was best for me. Shortly after dialysis, I was evaluated for a kidney transplant and found to be a good candidate. I was added to the transplant list. All of my family members were tested, but none were a match.

To stay on the transplant list, I had to do a monthly blood screening. I knew if it was God's will for me to have a transplant, he would provide an angel just for me.

The call came on August 28, 2011. My entire family quickly gathered themselves together for the great day—the day we traveled to Ann Arbor. Waiting had not been easy, but I knew it was God's plan. I waited patiently with a positive attitude and a will to do all that the doctor prescribed.

The surgery went smoothly; however, there were complications afterwards. Some were critical, but eventually they were resolved, and I was sent home. There were critical times after I went home, too, and I had to return to the hospital many times. When my condition improved, I went to University of Michigan Health System (UMHS) weekly, then biweekly, monthly, every three months, and, finally, yearly. I also see my local nephrologist twice yearly and get blood work monthly for signs of rejection and to monitor the level of medications in my blood.

I have many, many medications to take. The antirejection drug doesn't always agree with my system. One drawback is that my weight is uncontrollable due to the medication. I have experienced tremors, perspiration, and water retention as a result of the medications. I was also diagnosed with cancer.

I am so very grateful for the family who shared a part of their loved one with me. To God be the glory.

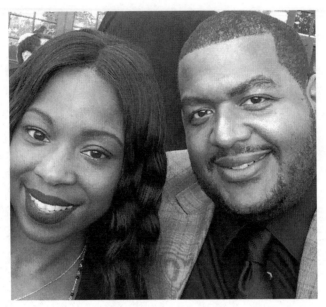

Elisa (left) and Justin (right)

# Justin's Story

Justin was diagnosed with hypertensive nephrosclerosis and received a transplant at 31 years old from a living donor.

It was August 2007 when I married my beautiful wife, Elisa. At the time, we were looking forward to getting away from reality and really enjoying our first vacation as husband and wife on a honeymoon cruise. The cruise lived up to our expectations, but I was sick on multiple occasions. Elisa and I thought it was seasickness or maybe trying different foods.

During that same winter, Elisa found out she was pregnant. I remember like it was yesterday. We were both excited and delivered the news to our families on Christmas Day that year. The excitement of expecting our first son was short-lived due to Elisa's morning sickness. I began to have a reaction to her sickness and became sick myself—at least, that is what I thought. Eventually Elisa's morning sickness passed, but I was still getting sick. I also began to get very bad headaches to the point that I went nights without sleep.

One day I walked into work taking the stairs like I normally do to the fifth floor, but this day was a little different. I had to stop on the third floor because I needed to catch my breath, which I never had to do before. I continued up the stairs very slowly until I reached my desk. I recall sitting at my desk for a couple of hours in a daze. Coworkers asked what was wrong and said I didn't look well. I wasn't feeling well, so I called my doctor and went to his office. I went through the normal routine of getting my temperature, pulse, and blood pressure checked.

They checked my blood pressure several times. The doctor said I needed to go to the emergency room because I was on the verge of a stroke with my blood pressure so high. Once I got to the emergency room, they took me back right away to perform several tests. It was that day, March 18, 2008, that I was diagnosed with kidney disease. When I woke up that morning, I never thought this day would change the rest of my life.

Things began to happen so fast. It was not until that evening that the doctors informed me my kidneys had failed to the point of no return. I started dialysis that same day while still at the hospital. They told me my condition was attributed to high blood pressure that was untreated for so long. I was devastated, shocked, scared, and just unsure what was in my future. Most of all, I felt like I let Elisa down. We had been married less than a year. She was three months pregnant at the time and, on top of that, we were purchasing a house. I never knew anybody on dialysis. Here I am, this big, strong guy who never had a fear in the world until I was put on dialysis.

Elisa spent that first day with me in the hospital. We listened to doctors and nurses. We asked questions and got answers but were still in disbelief and uncertain of what would happen next. Soon after Elisa left to get some rest, friends and family started showing up in the middle of the night. My parents and friends were all in shock at the news. The looks on their faces made me feel like I disappointed them all. I was thinking, "Why me? What did I do to deserve this? How did I let it get this bad?"

Before going home, I was instructed to go to the dialysis center where I would be receiving my treatments. I met the nurses, social worker, dietician, techs, and about thirty or so other people receiving dialysis treatments at the center.

That first year was the most difficult year of my life. My treatments were on Mondays, Wednesdays, and Fridays. I would leave work at 2 p.m. on my treatment days and would dialyze for almost six hours. Treatments were harder than anything I had ever done before. I'd sit there while this machine pulled pounds of fluid and toxins from my body. When I first started dialysis, there were days when I would lose up to 16 pounds of fluid. Those days were the most draining on my body. At times, I would barely be able to walk to my car to get home. I would go home at night exhausted. The next day I would still be very tired when I got up for work. It wasn't until the day after that I would feel better, but that was the day I had another treatment. This cycle continued, day after day, while having in-center dialysis treatment.

I did in-center dialysis treatment for a year and a half. There were many difficulties Elisa and I had to adjust to. Since I was leaving work early during those treatment days, there was a big decrease in pay. While on dialysis, I was painting, making updates, and moving into our new home. Elisa had our son, Braylen, that September and adjusting to a newborn's schedule was difficult. When Elisa first had Braylen, I recall leaving the hospital to go for a dialysis treatment. I was in graduate school as well but didn't attend my graduation to receive my master's degree because I had treatment at that time. Life continued to go on as I sat in a chair, day after day, and I could not accept why this had happened to me.

After being on dialysis for a year and a half, I decided to make an appointment to be evaluated for a kidney transplant. The team determined I needed to lose some weight before becoming a good candidate. After my evaluation appointment, I had another appointment with another doctor. To this day I cannot recall what doctor I saw nor why I was there. The appointment was at the Cancer Center. I checked in, sat, and waited. While waiting, I noticed I was in the children's area.

So I sat among families with children who had cancer. Some had lost their hair from chemotherapy treatments. Many of them were wearing masks. Some just sat with their parents.

The one thing I noticed was they were all smiling, having fun playing with toys, laughing, and giggling, and I was thinking, "Woe is me." Here I was, almost 30 at the time, upset, broken, continuously questioning God. Then I see these children who were facing life-threatening situations but acting like normal kids. My life changed that day. I truly feel and believe God was showing me something. I learned that day that having kidney failure and being on dialysis would not define me, and I had to change my attitude to overcome that.

After that day, I became motivated; I was not going to feel defeated any longer. I began to get involved in my treatments. My treatments became more manageable. Life began to turn around. I had finally accepted being on dialysis after more than a year and was determined not to let it hold me back any longer.

I began to inquire about performing dialysis at home; I wanted to get back to working full-time. I wanted to be more available to help Elisa with Braylen. I wanted to have fun with my family and friends. After some discussion and training, I was able to do dialysis at home. Home dialysis is exactly what I needed at the time. It allowed me to live a normal life again. I had to dialyze six days a week for only two hours a day. If I managed my fluids and diet, I could stay on this regimen for my home treatments, and I did. I would run my treatments before work and live the rest of my day like everybody else. Life felt normal again for the first time in a long time.

Life was moving in the right direction when I did my treatments at home but my ultimate goal was to get a kidney transplant. I was added to the transplant list but was still possibly looking at years before I'd be matched to a donor. My family had all been tested the year before, but none were a match. There was only one person who wanted to be tested but had not, and that was Elisa. She couldn't get tested because she had to wait a year after giving birth to Braylen. When the conversation came up, I did not want her to donate a kidney to me. I instantly thought the worst and didn't want anything to happen to her. She had already been through so much being by my side through it all. I'll admit I was stubborn at the time, but I felt like I had valid reasons. Finally, she convinced me that if a kidney would get me off dialysis and back home, then she wanted to be tested.

It turned out that Elisa was a good match to donate her kidney to me. We were shocked and elated about the news. We continued going through the transplant process until we had a transplant date scheduled for right after Thanksgiving. I was filled with so many different emotions for the entire month before the surgery. I was excited and happy that I may soon be off dialysis. On the other hand, the risk that something could happen to Elisa was troubling. I was on an emotional roller coaster that month. After many days and many hours of prayer, I turned it over to God because it was much bigger than us.

We finally came to the day of the surgery on December 21, 2011. I was tired that day with everything going through my mind, and I had overslept. Elisa and I arrived at the hospital early in the morning. The hospital was busy and crowded with doctors, nurses, patients, and family members. There was much nervousness and anticipation in the preoperative room, which was now empty, except for our family. There was a nice, peaceful moment before surgery. Elisa was soon taken back, and I followed shortly after. After surgery, I woke up and noticed Elisa to my left. I immediately asked if everything went well with her procedure, and the nurses confirmed it had. I was happy at that point because she was my priority. The nurses told me my own surgery had gone well and the kidney was already functioning.

After the surgery, Elisa spent a couple of days in the hospital and then went home for the rest of her recovery. She was back to work in just a couple of weeks. I stayed in the hospital during this time. I wasn't upset that I had to stay in the hospital during Christmas and on New Year's Day because I knew it was only a matter of time before I would be going home. It wasn't until early January that I was able to leave. I recall walking out of the hospital and feeling the wind hit my face, smelling the fresh air, and thinking I never thought I'd get to this point.

It took me a couple of months to recover after my kidney transplant, even though I felt much better immediately after the transplant. I thought about how long I had been sick, even since before dialysis; I felt like a new man. My first day back at work, coworkers were telling me how my eyes cleared up from being glassy and were white again. I didn't realize the change because it was normal to me. It felt amazing to have my life back again and not have to perform my daily dialysis treatments.

My health and kidney are doing very well six years later. I have to get blood work drawn monthly, and I see the kidney doctors yearly. The fact that I'm still being monitored gives me some comfort in case something were to happen. Elisa is healthy and has never had any setbacks. In fact, we had another son named Drew, who is three, and Braylen is now seven. My motivation is trying to stay healthy for them while also staying involved in the transplant community.

I am currently volunteering as a peer mentor. I go to dialysis centers in my area and speak with other patients who are on dialysis. I tell them my story and let them know I was in that chair receiving dialysis treatment not long ago. I answer questions they have about dialysis and the process of receiving a kidney transplant. Many of them are worried, just like I was about Elisa. They have loved ones who want to donate their kidneys, but they don't want anything to happen to those loved ones. I explain to them that it is a decision both parties have to make together.

Patients appreciate the time I spend talking with them. It is one thing to listen to a doctor or nurse who may have no idea what the patient is feeling, but to have the chance to listen to somebody who has been in their shoes goes a long way. I will continue to reach out and speak to patients. I will continue to be involved in discussions with doctors, nurses, and other staff about dialysis and my experience after kidney transplant. I want them to have all the tools and to share my experience with their patients.

I want to thank my family and friends for all of the encouragement and support. There were days and times when things were not going well, and a simple call or text message would do wonders for us. There were times when family would take me to doctor appointments or meet me there to keep me company. Some cooked us meals and some watched the children. I recall good friends taking me to the barber shop or picking up medication because I could not drive. They would take the trash out for me because I didn't have the strength to do it. I can go on and on about how much I appreciate them playing a part in helping me reach my ultimate goal.

I also want to thank all the dialysis techs, nurses, and doctors for seeing me through this process. I definitely could not have done this alone. They took the time to answer all my questions. They were all so patient with me during the hard times before I accepted dialysis. I still go back to my dialysis unit to visit with them. I let them know I appreciate them and could not be where I am today without them.

It was difficult writing this transplant story; we never want to go back to the difficult times in our lives and this surely was my most difficult. There were many dark days, moments when I questioned God and His purpose. The hardest impact was on those closest to me. Elisa was with me every step of the way. There were times she sat with me during treatments and times in the middle of the night when she would help me stretch because I would cramp up from treatment earlier that day. She spent weeks going through the home dialysis training. She carried so much of my burden and her own worries, all while having to work and take care of Braylen when he was first born. She would not allow me to give up. She needed me as much as I needed her.

I dedicate this story to the love of my life, Elisa. You really are an inspiration and you are so much stronger than you know. Thank you for believing in me, staying by my side, and pushing me not to settle.

As I look back now, this was not a setback, but more of a setup. God allows things to happen in our lives so we can get closer to Him. What I had to go through was unfortunate, but everybody has their own story. Everybody has a choice to try to get through tough times alone or, like me, give it all to God. There's no way I could have overcome this alone. I needed faith. Once again, God showed He is a healer to the sick, gives strength when you are weak, and is there (right on time) when you need Him. Thank you, God.

Editor's Note: Justin passed away, due to unrelated medical issues, shortly after submitting his story. His wife has given us permission to share his story. Justin was very excited to tell others about his experience. He was a great contributor to our Peer Mentor program and will be greatly missed.

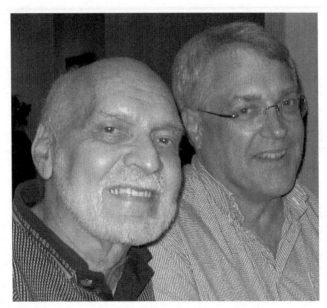

Jack (left) and Larry (right)

# Larry's Story

Larry donated at 55 years old to his Uncle Jack.

Most perfectly healthy people don't volunteer for major surgery. Living kidney donors are a different breed, though. I suppose we're altruistic. We want to help out. Donating your kidney is one of the most generous things you can do for another human being. But make no mistake: kidney donation is a major surgery. It causes you pain. It's inconvenient. It takes time to recuperate. Despite the pain, the inconvenience, and the downtime, I realize now that donating my spare kidney to my Uncle Jack was one of the most rewarding experiences of my life. If I had a third kidney, I'd give it to another dialysis patient. If you're considering kidney donation, I encourage you to think about giving yours to someone in need. Here is some advice.

## Don't Wait to Be Asked to Donate Your Kidney

Uncle Jack would never have asked for someone to give him a kidney. Most patients in need of a transplant feel the same way. They're reluctant to ask. Kidney donors need to step up.

My adventure in nephrology began at an unlikely spot—a Detroit Tigers baseball game. Each summer, men in our family have a tradition of attending a ballgame together for a boys' night out. On a hot summer night, a dozen years ago, Uncle Jack, my cousin Jimmy, and I were cheering on our Tigers. During the game, Uncle Jack mentioned that his doctors told him his kidneys were failing. He needed to start

51

hemodialysis. After that, there would be only one alternative to life on dialysis: a kidney transplant. The wait for a transplant from a deceased donor would be a long one: five to seven years. This was gut-wrenching news for Jimmy and me. We'd been there with Uncle Jack many years earlier when he'd survived a heart transplant. I didn't say anything about it during the game, but on my way home that night I wondered about a kidney transplant from a living donor. I wondered if I could be Uncle Jack's donor.

My wife, Linda, happens to be a nephrology nurse. Over the years, she has worked with many dialysis patients who received transplants from living donors. After talking it over, Linda said, "You have to do this! Life on dialysis can be pretty miserable. You'll be giving Uncle Jack his life back." I decided to inquire about whether I could donate a kidney to my uncle. I knew he would never ask, so I offered. When I called him, he was hesitant. After some persuading, Uncle Jack said he'd be willing to find out if we were a "match."

**Involve Your Loved Ones in Decision-Making**

My teenaged son asked, "What the hell are you thinking, Dad?" He and his older sisters were worried. I'd informed them that I was arranging to donate one of my kidneys to my uncle. Why, they asked, would I agree to undergo a major surgery when I was perfectly healthy?

"Surgery is for sick people," my son said.

"Well," I explained, "ever since your Grandpa Kloss died, Uncle Jack is the one man in this world I care about the most. Your grandma's baby brother—less than ten years older than me—is more like my big brother. Uncle Jack needs help and I think I can give it to him, with very little risk to myself."

As it turned out, I was right about that. Donating a kidney involves very little risk for the donor. I shared all this with my children because I wanted them to be involved with the process. I was curious to know what they were thinking. I wanted to reassure them. Gradually, they came around.

Today, as a Transplant Center Living Donor Mentor, I urge prospective donors to be mindful of loved ones who, like my children, may question their decisions to donate. Talk with them, encourage them to express their reservations, and reassure them that kidney donation is the right thing to do.

Uncle Jack and I made it through the transplant in great shape. Still, he and I traveled a long, difficult road on the way to our successful outcome.

## Contradictory Piece of Advice #1: Be Patient with the Process

After our initial match, the path to our transplant was filled with obstacles. It took well over a year to get to the operating room. On three or four occasions, Uncle Jack became very ill and very anemic. Every time he was hospitalized, he was given a blood transfusion. Each transfusion was, in effect, a "mini-transplant," where cells from someone else's body were introduced into Uncle Jack's body. His immune system produced new antibodies as it reacted to a blood transfusion. This meant he and I might no longer be a match. After each transfusion, we had to wait ninety days for the antibodies to be produced. Then, time after time, we began the matching process all over again. I grew impatient. More than once, I expressed my frustration to the Transplant Center staff. Finally, following delay after delay, our transplant happened.

**Contradictory Piece of Advice #2: Be Impatient with the Process**

I encourage potential donors to be the squeaky wheel when dealing with the Transplant Center. I invite them to reach out with concerns and to question delays. The center where I volunteer arranges nearly a hundred transplants with living donors each year. That is many balls to keep in the air at one time. Sometimes prospective donors wonder whether their transplants have been shoved to a back burner. If they feel that way I tell folks, "Don't hesitate. Pick up the phone or send an email. Contact the medical professionals at your transplant program." It really is true that squeaky wheels get greased.

**Expect Some Pain and Overestimate Your Recovery Period**

Uncle Jack's transformation after the transplant was incredible. I was amazed to learn that, like many recipients, his new kidney began producing urine while he was still on the operating table. His energy and color returned almost immediately. His jaundiced eyes and yellow skin were gone. At last, he was untethered from his dialysis machine. He and my aunt were ecstatic. My kidney-nurse wife was ecstatic. I, on the other hand, felt like I'd been run over by a truck.

Removing my kidney required about a four-inch incision through my core muscles next to my belly button. I never realized how often we use these muscles. Climbing a flight of stairs was nearly impossible. Shifting in my chair, rolling over in bed, and especially defecating, were real struggles.

Every donor's experience is different, of course. In my case, I hated the narcotics prescribed for my pain. They caused bizarre dreams, and when I was awake, the walls sometimes looked like they were moving. I probably weaned myself off the narcotics sooner than I should have, but I preferred a moderate level of pain over the drug-induced weirdness. Regular acetaminophen took the edge off the pain and, gradually, it faded away. After recuperating for six weeks, I felt as good as new.

## If You're Not One Already, Become a Water Drinker

Healthcare professionals say it's a good idea to be well hydrated when you report for surgery. Drink at least two liters of water every day, they say. Pain medication, combined with your reluctance to move much after a nephrectomy, can contribute to constipation. And being constipated can cause real problems. It's critically important to take the stool softeners that will be prescribed when you go home from the hospital. Straining in the bathroom can interfere with your recuperation by causing a hernia. The last thing you'll want to do after kidney removal will be to return to the operating room for a hernia repair.

Long before my surgery, I made sure I drank plenty of water each day. I filled an empty, two-liter, soda-pop bottle with water every morning and set it in the refrigerator. I made sure it was empty every night before bed. I was well hydrated when I arrived for the transplant surgery.

## Lean on Your Support Network and Plan on Making a Full Recovery

Transplant centers screen potential kidney donors very carefully. They want to make sure the donor will make it through the transplant experience without any adverse effects. You'll receive the most thorough physical exam of your life. If you are approved to donate a kidney, you can be confident you're one of the healthiest people walking around. You are not superhuman, however. You'll need a strong support network to help you during your recovery. Let them do the housework, the grocery shopping, and all the lifting—heavy or otherwise. To protect you from a hernia, you'll be restricted from lifting anything heavier than ten pounds (about the weight of a gallon of milk).

When you begin feeling better, it's tempting to start overdoing it. It's important to listen to your body when it tells you you've exerted yourself enough and it's time to rest. If you take it slow, your recovery should be smooth and uneventful.

## Life with One Kidney

I volunteer with Michigan Medicine as a Living Donor Peer Mentor. One of the most common questions I get is, "How is your life different since you donated a kidney?" The first few times I heard this, I had a hard time coming up with an answer. Once I had recovered from the transplant surgery, my life returned to normal. Nothing seemed different. Later, I realized there is one important difference. Prior to the transplant, I was very "hit or miss" about getting yearly physicals. Now, I follow the Transplant Center's advice: I have my kidney function checked every year at a physical exam. Two years ago, my physical uncovered something suspicious with my prostate. It was cancer. Thanks to early detection, I am now cancer-free. I tell people that, in a way, donating a kidney saved my life.

## The Second Happiest Thing

A few years ago, my younger daughter gave birth to our first grandchild. As she lay there glowing in her hospital bed, I said, "You know, many things that happen in hospitals aren't very happy. The absolute happiest thing that happens in a hospital is the birth of a healthy baby."

"It sure is," she said.

Then I added, "And do you know the second happiest thing that happens in a hospital? A successful kidney transplant from a living donor."

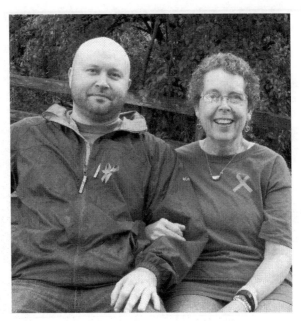

Kevin (left) and Margo (right)

# Margo's Story

Margo was diagnosed with hypertensive nephrosclerosis and received a transplant at 62 years old from a living donor.

Life is always an adventure. I've certainly had quite an adventure with chronic kidney disease (CKD). Despite the impact on my life and the lives of my family, I am thankful for this adventure. I've learned so much, my faith has grown, and I've met people I wouldn't have otherwise. My life is rich in blessings!

One year prior to being diagnosed with CKD in 2005, I went for a regular checkup with my internist. My blood pressure was higher than normal but I chalked it up to being nervous about seeing my doctor. My doctor told me that my blood pressure was too high and prescribed hypertension medication. I started the medication and didn't think any more about it. I thought medication alone would take care of it. It was not long until I found out that ignorance is not bliss.

Everything changed in 2006 when I returned to my doctor for my yearly checkup. She was concerned that my kidney function was at 29 percent and referred me to a local nephrologist. Further testing by the nephrologist confirmed that I was in Stage 4 kidney disease with a glomerular filtration rate (GFR) of 29. To say that I was shocked was an understatement. It was a lot to take in, especially since I had no symptoms except for the hypertension, which was being treated. I was so thankful that my nephrologist answered the many questions I had about kidney disease and hypertension. Now I could keep myself as healthy as possible. I also found resources such as the National Kidney

Foundation and the Renal Support Network, which helped educate me about kidney disease, gave me hope, and eased my anxiety.

I am fortunate to have a very loving and supportive family. I was very matter-of-fact in explaining my chronic kidney disease diagnosis. I also explained how my nephrologist felt confident I could have a good quality of life at Stage 4 CKD and that it could be many years before I would need to look into dialysis or a kidney transplant. It wasn't long afterwards that our son, Kevin, told me he had researched kidney disease. He also said that when I needed to have a kidney transplant, he wanted to donate one to me. His love and generosity floored me. It still does to this day.

I stayed in Stage 4 CKD for eight years, until 2014 when my GFR slid into Stage 5. My hypertension had gotten harder to control, and two additional hypertensive medications had been added. I had more fatigue, but I could not tell if it was from my kidney disease, getting older, all of the hard work I do on our farm, or a combination of everything. Over the course of the summer, however, I started feeling worse with even more fatigue. I was feeling cold even in the heat of summer and I had a funny, metallic taste in my mouth. I knew my kidney function was getting worse.

I was not surprised when my nephrologist said it was time for me to take dialysis classes and to be evaluated for a kidney transplant. Taking the dialysis classes and going through the kidney transplant evaluation process made it very real that my body was very sick and needed a new treatment plan. I was thankful there were treatment options for my CKD.

It was then that Kevin said he still wanted to be my donor and would even go through paired donation if we weren't a match. His desire to be a donor was such an act of love; it gave me hope for the possibility of a future of improved health.

After I was accepted into the kidney transplant program and put on the organ transplant waitlist, Kevin went through the donor evaluation process. Both of us were relieved, and I was thankful, when we found out he was a match. However, he couldn't donate a kidney to me unless he lost 30 pounds. He was so worried that I would need dialysis before he lost the weight. Kevin showed his determination to be my donor by losing the weight by the spring of 2015.

In late March 2015, four months after being put on the waitlist and, thankfully, still holding my own physically with no dialysis, there were many tears of joy when Kevin called to tell me he had lost the weight needed. He asked if May 1, 2015, sounded like a good date for our surgery. I was speechless at first and, after absorbing what he said, told him over and over how thankful I was. My husband and I said many prayers giving thanks that day for the beautiful hope of improved health that Kevin's future gift of a kidney would give me. Our whole family rejoiced and was thankful for Kevin's upcoming gift of life for me. Everyone in the family discussed how each of them could help Kevin and me during and after our surgeries. It was amazing the amount of support Kevin and I received from our family, both during our hospital stay and during post-surgical recovery.

When I look back at the six months prior to receiving Kevin's kidney, however, that time frame seemed to move slowly. I continued to feel worse and had even greater fatigue. I really am fortunate that it was a short time waiting for a kidney, especially given the waitlist time of five to seven years. I am thankful I didn't have any hospitalizations that would have delayed the transplant and didn't end up needing emergency dialysis.

My life changed forever when I received Kevin's kidney on May 1, 2015. When I woke up in recovery, my first question was to ask how Kevin was doing. Once I was told he was recovering well, I asked about my surgery. I was so thankful to learn that everything went well and that I had a big, beautiful, well-functioning, and young kidney that urinated right away. I was amazed at how much better I felt after I was moved to my hospital room. The crushing fatigue had eased, I was no longer freezing cold, and the toxic taste in my mouth that had bothered me for over four months had disappeared. I never dreamed I would feel as good as I did so quickly with my new kidney. I lovingly named it the Whiz Kid. I praised God and was thankful for the skill of both of our surgeons and their teams that resulted in successful surgeries for Kevin and me.

Kevin's recovery was more challenging than mine. He had pain from surgery that took about three weeks to heal. He had a great attitude and told me not to worry as he knew that each day he was one day closer to feeling like himself. Recently he told me he doesn't feel any different with one kidney, and he is glad that he donated. It meant a lot to him to see how my quality of life has improved with a kidney transplant. He doesn't see himself as a hero, but Kevin is definitely my hero.

I will always be very thankful for my kidney transplant team, who have given me the best of care and educated me on how to take care of my Whiz Kid from the beginning.

I had a few bumps along my kidney transplant journey, such as a blood clot three weeks after surgery that required treatment for six months. I had low white-blood-cell counts that ended with steroids being added to my transplant medications. I had a diagnosis of hydronephrosis one year post-transplant. With each challenge, my transplant nephrologist developed a successful treatment plan. I have complete confidence in the care I received at the University of Michigan Transplant Center. It is so comforting to know that my transplant team is only a phone call away. I am hearing-impaired and use cochlear implants to hear. I appreciate the extra effort my kidney transplant team takes to make sure my communication needs are met. My kidney transplant team has become a part of my extended family; they want me to have the healthiest life possible, just as my family and I do. It is greatly appreciated.

I am aware that my kidney transplant is a treatment. I want to take great care of my Whiz Kid so that he lasts for many, many years. This transplant is such a precious gift. For me, putting my medications in a weekly pill organizer and setting a 9 a.m. and 9 p.m. alarm on my phone and activity tracker is so important since it is so easy to get distracted. Staying hydrated is vital, and at mealtimes I think about how much water I've drunk throughout the day so that by evening I make sure I've had my daily water quota. My activity tracker has helped to keep me motivated to exercise 40-60 minutes a day. When the weather allows, I enjoy walking for exercise. I have hand weights and an exercise bike for indoor exercise. Exercise with friends is a lot more fun. I love going to yoga, line dancing, and tai chi with friends when I can.

I think my biggest challenge lies in healthy eating. It is a struggle to keep my hunger at bay. I have to be very aware of what I'm eating each day. I also have some minor hand tremors that come and go from one of my medications. I had some hair loss for the first ten months after kidney transplant; my hair is thinner than it was before transplant. Those side effects are minor compared to the blessings of improved health. Keeping myself grounded with a good sense of humor is key to managing them.

Throughout my transplant journey, I've felt it is important to teach my family and friends about how I need to take care of my kidney, pay attention to health concerns, and keep my lifestyle clean and safe to avoid infections. I want them to understand when they see me using hand sanitizer, avoiding salad bars at restaurants, staying away from people who are sick, taking my transplant medications on time, and other daily tasks to keep my kidney and me as healthy as possible. My family and friends are another part of my kidney transplant team. I also think my CKD-to-kidney-transplant journey has helped my family and friends to be more aware of their own health and how precious good health is.

Having CKD and receiving this most precious kidney transplant has taught me so much. I am thankful for the lessons I have learned. Leaning on my faith and practicing perseverance, joy, and how to maintain a positive attitude during my kidney transplant journey has been, and continues to be, important for my physical and mental health. I've learned to see myself as part of a team that includes my transplant team, my local nephrologist, family, friends, and fellow kidney transplant donors and recipients who have become mentors and friends.

Together, we all work to keep me and the Whiz Kid as healthy as possible. I have learned to rejoice at the smallest joys that occur each day. The joy of being outside, enjoying the beautiful views of our apple and peach orchards while I walk; having small conversations with my husband without feeling fatigued; being able to play with my young grandchildren; sharing laughter while being with friends and family. All of the many everyday life moments fill me with boundless gratitude for my life with this beautiful kidney. I always have joy and thankfulness for each precious day.

I have so much hope for the future with my Whiz Kid. When I look back at how far kidney transplants have come in the past 50 years, I truly believe that future technology and advances in kidney transplant care and medications for kidney transplant recipients will continue to evolve, which is so exciting. I want to keep myself as healthy as possible so that I will be able to take advantage of whatever new treatments or medications come along to help me continue enjoying this incredible life of mine. Should any serious health- or kidney-related challenges occur in the future, I am confident that my kidney transplant team, the support of my family and friends, as well as my faith and positive attitude will lead to the best outcome possible, whatever the challenge.

As my transplant nephrologist once told me, "We didn't give you a kidney transplant to make your life difficult and isolating, but to give you another chance of living." I am living life to the fullest with my Whiz Kid!

I feel so blessed.

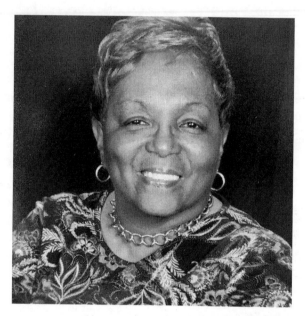

Marilyn

# Marilyn's Story

Marilyn was diagnosed with type 2 diabetes and received a transplant at 61 years old from a deceased donor.

My battle with diabetes led to my chronic kidney disease (CKD). It seemed that every time I went to my nephrologist, my kidney function had decreased. It made it to CKD 5. My nephrologist advised me that since the organ transplant waitlist was so long, I should get on the list early. I was never on dialysis. I thought, "Oh my, I am going to have to quit my job in order to go to dialysis." I never told friends and barely touched on the information with my family.

I decided to be on the list at the insistence of my doctor. I was on two different transplant lists (in two different states), thinking the University of Michigan Health System (UMHS) would have the longest waiting time. All of a sudden, one morning, after about three years, my telephone rang and it was UMHS saying, "We have a kidney for you." I was very excited in one sense. In another sense, I was thinking, "Suppose everything doesn't match, I might not be a recipient." Fortunately, after getting to the hospital, everything matched and I was on my way.

I did not seek a living donor. I kept my spirits up by praying and engaging with family and people at my job. I did not let anything get me down.

I managed my health by staying upbeat, knowing my life had changed from the struggle of many years. I am a strong person, so I would suggest to a person considering a kidney transplant to stay strong. Some people cannot survive without others; I am a person who can.

I did finally tell my family how sick I really was. I couldn't stand to smell food or cologne. For two weeks, I would only eat fresh peaches. I lost 15 pounds during this time. Now I can eat anything and my complexion is very nice.

Whether you should tell your family and friends about your kidney problems is something you will have to decide. I did not really share until I had the transplant. Of course they all asked why I didn't say something. My reply was, "You could not make me feel better, and I didn't want you to worry."

The people I was assigned to for post-transplant care were Dr. S. and Nurse T. They are the best—caring, understanding, and excellent at staying in touch. I had never really had a major surgery before, but it was not bad for me. I think I was so thankful to have a new lease on life that I did not allow myself to be negative about anything.

After receiving the transplant, my quality of life really changed. I faced some problems with my lower back, but I see my future as bright. My complexion lightened as though I was a new person. I had more energy, my appetite was better, and I was no longer sick to my stomach. I was very upbeat and did not require a long healing period. I am basically a new person with a new life ahead.

Author's Note: This is dedicated to my husband, Jimmy, and to our family. Thank you for all the support. You never knew how sick I was. You didn't know because I never really shared that with you. I did not want you to worry. All you really saw was my very dark complexion.

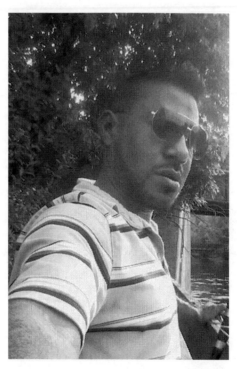

Miguel

# Miguel's Story

Miguel was diagnosed with hypertensive nephrosclerosis and received a transplant at 34 years old from a deceased donor.

I was 14 years old when I decided to leave my home country of Mexico without measuring the consequences of what could happen to me. Family problems came along, causing me to move out from my grandparent's home in Mexico. I left a note on the table explaining why I could no longer live there and thanking them for everything. Leaving my best wishes and blessings, the last words on the note were, "God has given you a heart and for every good act, He will bless you twice as much. I know my parents in Heaven are thankful for your help."

I went to the United States to live with a friend in California. At the time, everything was going well, but reality hit as soon as I was diagnosed with kidney problems at 19 years old. It never crossed my mind at that age I could suffer from kidney problems, and I could not imagine how I was going to deal with it. To me it felt like, as we say in my country, "como un valdo de agua fria," which means, "like a bucket of cold water." I felt paralyzed when I heard the doctor say what he found. It hit me so hard that tears started falling down my cheeks, but I couldn't feel them. I was completely shocked.

The doctor touched my shoulder and said, "Everything will be alright."

At that moment, my life had taken a 180-degree turn. I had no clue what I was going to do or how I was going to get over it. I had no family when I needed them the most; they ignored me and turned their backs. Being alone, that's when I started to remember my grandpa's words, "True friends are found at the hospital or in jail."

Lots of questions crossed my mind. Who was going to help me? Would anyone give me their support? All my family was in Mexico. How would I pay for rent, food, or medicine? Just as I thought all was lost, God sent me an angel. Thanks to him, I was able to survive for a while. But I'll talk more about him later.

I was fired from my last job because of my condition. They started taking hours away from my schedule, then told me work was very slow and I had to leave. I had a little bit of money saved, and the first few nights I would sleep in my car. Every day I would go out looking for a job, but it was hard because I also had to go to my dialysis appointments.

I like working in construction, so that's the type of job I was looking for. I found someone who would hire me, but I would have to work late nights and I couldn't do that because I had a treatment to follow. Potential employers would notice the fistula in my hand and would ask what was happening. I just told them it was a scar. I was trying to hide the fact that I had a health problem, but eventually I had to tell the truth. One day, after I found a new job, I was taken to the office to talk to the manager. He told me I could no longer work for them in my condition because if something were to happen to me, the company would have problems. For the second time, I had to stop working. I felt really sad and my self-esteem was failing. I tried to be positive about finding another job, but sometimes I felt lost.

It wasn't just hard with my jobs, but also with the places I would rent because sometimes I would be late with my payments, and I would have to leave and sleep in my car for days. I would knock on so many doors and none of them would open, but I kept believing that one of them would. I could see how people would look at me, leaving me again with no hope of finding a job or a place to live. I would walk away feeling something heavy on my shoulders and my feet couldn't take any more steps.

I got in my car and immediately started crying. I knew I was running out of money and didn't know if I would find another job in time. Many people told me just to go back to Mexico, and I would tell them that if I could, I would, but if I left in my condition, I wouldn't live much longer. When I talked to my grandparents in Mexico, I would always tell them not to worry about me. It was clear to them that I wasn't telling the truth. My voice would break and tears would fall again.

I lost my dad when I was three years old and my mom when I was six. Life started taking a toll on me in the hardest way, which is why I decided not to tell my family members what was going on with my health. However, I knew I wasn't going to be able to cover the sun with one finger. I would have to tell them at some point.

I kept looking for a job but had no luck. I ended up selling my car in order to rent a place to live. Honestly, sleeping in a car is not comfortable but at least I had somewhere to stay. I never wanted to sleep on the streets. For now, I would go and stand outside stores like Home Depot or Lowe's to see if anyone that went there needed a worker. I never imagined myself in this situation.

Dialysis is not easy. It takes much of your time and energy. It makes you feel weak because you have to limit your liquid intake and follow a strict diet. There are so many foods you can't have, and I had to adjust to that on top of being discriminated against. I felt lonely and hopeless. The money I had from selling my car was eventually gone and

I still couldn't find a job. Sometimes I would work three days a week, sometimes only one, or none at all. I was totally defeated. I always tried to think positively, telling myself I would be victorious.

Next thing I knew, five years had gone by, but everything was the same. It was hard to live that way, doing my dialysis treatments and not having anyone to support me. Thankfully, I was sure my parents were watching over me and sending me strength. I had no car, no job, and was in a tough situation, which worried me even more. The last place I was renting was taken away from me. I got home one day to find that the landlord had changed the lock and, again, I was homeless. I found my things outside in the yard. I asked for a plastic bag to carry my things. It made me feel miserable but I had more spirit to keep going. Back in Mexico, I had people who cared about me. I was always thinking about my grandparents and I thought of seeing them again.

I knew I had to keep fighting. I spent many cold and sad nights sleeping on the streets. These were dangerous nights because living on the streets of California is not safe. I eventually found a homeless shelter and spent some time there, but after a few days, I decided to leave because of the gang activity and theft. I was out on the streets again for at least three weeks, still trying to find a job. I did many things that never would have crossed my mind, like looking in trash cans to find some food because I had to take my medicine and I couldn't do it on an empty stomach. What was I going to do if I couldn't find a job? Everywhere I would go, I felt discriminated against. Employers would tell me to wait for their call, obviously never paying attention to me when I would tell them I didn't have a phone and there was no way for them to contact me. It breaks my heart to remember all those things.

I felt tired of having no place to live, no job, and a body and mind that were just exhausted. I arrived at the park that had been a home to me and laid on the same bench I always had. I don't know what happened next, but when I woke up, I was at the hospital and two days had gone by. I asked what had happened, and the nurse told me security came to ask me to leave but I wasn't responding when they tried to wake me up. The guy called an ambulance, and I was taken to the hospital. I just kept thinking about my family and I cried once more. The nurse asked if anyone could come pick me up, and I just smiled. She stared at me and asked why I was smiling. I replied, "If I had someone, do you think they would have found me sleeping at the park?" She offered me an apology and told me she couldn't help me find a job but she knew where I could live for now.

When I left the hospital four days later, I was taken to my new home. The hospital paid for temporary housing for people who had no place to go. I was so happy because the hospital said they would pay for everything. When I felt better, I went back to looking for a job with the best attitude ever, always praying God would keep me safe and healthy. Every day is a new day to thank the Lord for a new opportunity of waking up, because death is the only thing with no solution. Some days I would find some work, and some days I was not so lucky. I would stay long hours, hoping someone would show up needing workers. One day, a very elegant car approached with a lady driving. She walked up to me and touched my shoulder. When I looked up to her she handed me five dollars. I offered to wash her car but she told me to just take the money. I began to cry and said, "God bless you; thanks for this."

I have gone through many things, but I still think life is beautiful. Once I found a steady job, I started saving money so I could live somewhere else—start living a "normal" life—and keep following my treatments until I could have my transplant. I was anxious for that moment to come so I could finally be okay. I wanted to feel good about myself again.

Dialysis is something that needs to be followed and should be taken seriously. It is not good to drink too many liquids because your kidney is not functioning well. This was something I could not understand and would not follow. I was really stubborn, but I had to learn to do as the doctor said. At one point, the treatment stopped working. My feet and arms were swollen and I went to the hospital right away. When I got there, I was given a dose of morphine for the pain and I felt like my whole body was asleep. After a while, I went to sleep and the nurse decided to put me in a more comfortable position. Shortly after, I was screaming for help. I just could not breathe. I felt like a fish taken out of water, until I collapsed.

I woke up eight days later. I was tied up with a big tube in my mouth. When I asked what happened, they told me I had been in a coma because of all the liquid I had in my body. The doctor told me I was lucky the water did not touch my heart. He explained to me that when liquid gets to the heart, it starts to fill up and stops working. After this incident, I had learned my lesson. I had to learn the hard way to follow instructions very carefully. I was given a second chance to do it right. I had to be extremely careful with what I would drink and eat.

I met a guy at work, someone I could truly call my friend. He did something I will never forget. Barely knowing me, he offered me his house and was really nice to me. He was a true friend. I thought all my problems were over, but then I felt my depression and, again, I was taken to the hospital for two weeks. I was in a room all alone without any access to the outside world. I would scream so they would let me out but the more I yelled, the more I knew they would refuse. They thought I was crazy, so I had to show them I knew what I was doing. I wasn't crazy, I was just depressed.

Those two weeks were hard. They finally moved me to another room with a big window and a great view. I only had to spend three days there before I was told to go back home. I called my manager to let him know what had happened and to ask if I still had my job. They just told me to get a doctor's note and I would have my job back. I thanked the Lord and my manager for giving me my job again. When I got back to my job, I saw my friend. He gave me a big hug and asked me if I was ready to go home with him. I was speechless. I knew God would always bless him and his family for all their help. His family treated me as one of them.

I left California to live near my aunt and cousins who moved from Mexico to Michigan. I was blessed to find out I would be able to get my transplant here after 15 years of being in treatment. I would have the opportunity to recover and start a new life. I was so happy and I felt that God had listened to my prayers.

I hope to someday go back to my country and see my grandparents again. They are all I have and for many years they were like my parents after my real parents died. I remember when I had to do my treatment, I felt like a dog on a leash because I was so restricted. It was hard for me to move around, but now everything is so much easier.

Please never give up no matter how hard life gets. Hard work pays off. Feel proud of everything you do with all your heart. I hope this story was able to inspire each and every one of you to keep going forward.

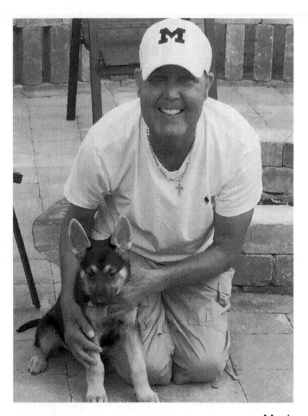

Mark

# Mark's Story

Mark was diagnosed with type 1 diabetes and received two transplants, one at 27 years old from a deceased donor and one at 45 years old from a living donor.

Freedom is a powerful word. It is used often by many, interpreted differently by most, at times misunderstood, and often taken for granted. The word "freedom" is all-encompassing. It is regularly craved and sought out, yet can simultaneously be given away. Below is my story involving struggles; harsh realities; and the power of positive thinking, inner-peace, and true selflessness. It is also a story about the gift of freedom—what it means to me and how important it is. It's about two people, one a perfect stranger with a giving soul and the other an angel walking this earth, who gifted me with the ultimate freedom—my life.

I was nine years old when first diagnosed. I knew my older sister, Cheryl, had been given the label, and although I had witnessed her struggles, nothing could have fully prepared me for the life changes that the diagnosis would sentence me to. It was type 1 diabetes, a condition in which one's pancreas does not produce the amount of insulin required to keep the human body and organs functioning properly. I knew treatment was possible to help prevent symptoms, but I quickly learned that my childhood would be very different from most of the other children I grew up with.

Shots, shots, and more shots is much of what I remember in the beginning. As a young diabetic, insulin shots were a necessity and I had to give myself four of them per day for many years. The average childhood most people experience was out of the question for me.

Strenuous activity posed a problem, swapping food at lunches was a no-no, and sleepovers were usually not an option. I did not want to tell my friends about my condition as I feared they might have thought differently of me. I also never wanted to be a burden or pitied by anyone. Therefore, most of my friends at the time had no idea I was giving myself shots daily while struggling with a strict exercise regimen and a diet that was very difficult to stick to, especially as a child. It was never easy, that is for sure. I remember always thinking positively about the future. I attribute that way of thinking to my amazing support system. Thanks to the close family and friends who stuck by my side and encouraged me along the way, I look back upon my childhood very fondly, despite the diabetes.

The teenage years soon came and I found myself in more of a groove, so to speak. Life was not perfect, and I still tried to hide my diabetes, but at 16 I had a good job, a car, and girlfriends. What more could a teenage boy ask for? Spreading my wings in those years meant trying new things, exploring and experimenting with friends, making both good and bad decisions along the way, and enjoying as much of my youth as possible. I wanted to do all the things my friends were doing. I wanted to go to parties and eat and drink whatever sounded good. It was easy to sometimes convince myself at that age that just the insulin shots would be enough, and I would be just fine. Time after time, however, I would learn a difficult lesson the hard way and send my parents into panic mode when my sugar would drop or spike. I wound up in the hospital for almost a week at age 16, with sugar levels through the roof, and I was immediately snapped back into reality about the necessity of taking care of myself. I made it through those years, and although I can look back upon them now and smile, I did not come out unscathed. My body was not happy, but still, I remained positive.

I turned 21 years of age, finally able to legally drink alcohol, but instead of doing what most 21 year olds I knew were doing (going out to the bars and drinking with friends), I had to do the opposite. I was told by my doctor that year that I would need a transplant at some point if I ever wanted a normal life again, and I would need to abruptly make some serious lifestyle changes. I had to quit drinking alcohol altogether and be much more careful about my diet and exercise. My health was deteriorating quickly, and it felt as though everything came to a halt. The worst part about hearing such news in that moment was feeling as though my life had only just begun.

At that time, I was working many hours managing a well-known shoe store and making more money than most people my age. I was dating a woman I was starting to fall for and making plans for a future that would hopefully involve a wife, children, and success—among many other great things. I started to feel very sorry for myself. It was a very low point in time for me. Not only did I quickly learn who my true friends were, but at the same time, I pushed certain people away because I feared hurting them in the long run. It is a very difficult feeling to describe, but in a certain way, I felt like damaged goods. I continued to work, but my life was changing rapidly in all other areas, most especially my health.

Over the course of the next five years, I experienced numerous difficulties with my health. When a person's organs are slowly shutting down, their physical appearance changes, fatigue sets in, and even though it is hard to get out of bed in the morning, sleep doesn't come easily. I started losing weight rapidly. I remember being a measly 90 pounds at one point. I began to lose my vision. After seeing a retinal specialist and having multiple laser surgeries to help improve my eyesight, I was still struggling. A surgery might help temporarily, but never for long. I will never forget the day I lost vision completely in my right eye as I was driving. I was 25 years old at the time and on my way to work.

From that point forward, I was forced to come out about my diabetes with everyone. I could no longer drive to and from work. My parents were amazing during that time, taking turns driving me and trying to keep my spirits up. Without the support and encouragement of my family, I don't think I would have been able to manage. I saw many different doctors over the next year.

At age 25, I went to see a nephrologist/kidney specialist. After running several tests, I was told there was not much time left. If I wanted to have a life again, I needed to start dialysis immediately and be put on the list to receive a donor kidney as soon as possible. I knew I was in trouble at that point, and although I will admit I was scared—having already witnessed my sister who had gone through the transplant process a few years prior—I was doing my best to remain positive.

I was told to call three different hospitals to see what they could offer for transplants. I called two local hospitals and the University of Michigan Health System (UMHS). The first two said they would need evaluations prior to putting me on a list. UMHS asked what caused my kidney failure, and I told them I was a type 1 diabetic. They immediately asked if I would be willing to receive a pancreas and kidney transplant together, simultaneously, and I knew right then, that would be the hospital for me.

I scheduled a day and time to have an all-day evaluation at UMHS, and at the same time, I also became an official dialysis patient.

The medical team installed a port in my neck, created a fistula by tying my artery and vein together, and began the treatment of hemodialysis.

Unfortunately, it did not work. Each time the nurse would attach me to the machine, I would lose consciousness. After several attempts to no avail, I ultimately had to be put on a different form of dialysis—known as peritoneal—which uses the peritoneum in a person's abdomen to exchange fluid and substances within the blood. My mother had to be trained to perform it properly at home four times per day. As much as it was difficult for me, I am quite certain for my mother it was complete torture caring for and witnessing her son being in such pain and verging on death. My condition was slowly causing my organs to fail and, I must admit, I was in pretty rough shape. But I did my best to remain positive.

In and out of the hospital was my life. Tests, tests, and more tests became my normal. Evaluations are necessary when on a transplant list, as there are times when a person will not qualify to receive an organ. During this difficult, painful, and discouraging time in my life, one particular instance sticks out in my memory above many.

It was a day spent in the hospital, and I was in a mode of self-pity. I remember thinking to myself, "Why me," and asking God what I did to deserve such a sentence? I was walking through the cafeteria and remember looking directly at a table nearby, at which three young children sat, eating their food while smiling and laughing with each other. One of them was hooked up to a machine with several tubes running to and from her body. The other two were without hair, extremely pale, and frail. I stopped dead in my tracks and had an overwhelming feeling of guilt. I watched those precious children enjoying each other's company in even the most difficult of times and decided I was all done feeling sorry for myself. From that point forward, I made a vow to myself that I would do my best to never complain again and instead be grateful for the life I had been given. I had no clue at the time, but I would soon learn that I would have so much more life to be thankful for.

On July 17, 1993, one of my closest friends was having a graduation/ birthday celebration, and I had conjured up the energy to make it there and show my support. I had to be picked up and dropped off because my vision was so terrible. I have since been told that my two close friends looked at each other after dropping me off at home and said this was probably the last time they would see me alive. I'm glad I did not know that at the time, because I was still in a positive mood and was not giving up.

On July 19, the phone rang and I answered. They asked how quickly I could make it to the hospital, a pancreas and kidney was on its way. A 19-year-old young man had died in a car crash and generously elected to be an organ donor. I was in shock. So many emotions ran through me, I cannot begin to describe all of them. I felt sorrow for the young man losing his life and the grief his family must be going through yet a huge sense of relief and excitement that I was soon going to receive a second chance at my own life. I told the person on the other end I was sure we could leave right away and be there within the hour. I hung up the phone in disbelief. My mom, also in disbelief, thought I was messing with her at first, until she saw the look on my face. We headed out the door in a flash and made it to the hospital by 11 a.m. Shortly after 12 a.m. on the 20th, I had a new kidney and pancreas. I woke up feeling a new sense of hope. Although I knew recovery would not be easy, I was prepared to take on whatever came my way.

Postoperative recovery was pretty rough, and the difficulties resulting from my body reacting to its new organs made it even worse. I will not lie and say it was a walk in the park by any stretch of the imagination. There is a reason many people choose to stay on dialysis for years, refusing to have transplant surgery, and although I personally would always choose the transplant route over a lifetime of dialysis, I have always respected the choices of others. I was in the hospital for about two months with a high fever and trouble with the pancreas.

After being discharged in September, I was feeling pretty good. My energy level had increased, and my coloring was almost back to normal.

I also had a vitrectomy surgery performed to help remove some of the bleeding blood vessels behind my eyes that had caused my vision to deteriorate, and I will never forget the moment I could see again. Lying in the hospital bed prior to my release, with my dad in a chair beside me watching a ball game, I looked up and said what the score was out loud, and the look on my dad's face was priceless. All in all, things were looking up until November of 1993.

Two months after being discharged, my body started severely rejecting my organs, and the original antirejection medication I was put on was no longer effective. I was given a medicine that was the epitome of all ruthless medications in hopes of stopping the rejection. The nurses and doctors warned me it was a drug that would make me more sick than anything I had ever experienced, and they were not kidding. I thought I would be fine, as I figured I had been in enough pain before to handle anything.

To this day, I cannot remember a time when I felt more sick than I felt for those days following that medication entering my system. One would have thought I had ingested pure poison by the way my body reacted but, amazingly, it worked and ultimately stopped the rejection. Yet again, the doctors and nurses at UMHS were incredible during all of it. I truly cannot say enough about the staff in that hospital.

I had about four good years following the rejection ordeal and began working at one of the big three automotive companies, living life to the fullest. Unfortunately, once your body goes through such stress with diabetes and organ failure, nothing is ever quite the same. Blood circulation can already be a major issue for all diabetics. After a long day at work, I noticed a blister on my toe. Instead of healing, it progressively worsened until my entire toe was black and my foot was on its way. I went to the nearest hospital, hoping they could fix whatever was preventing the blood flow to my foot. The angiogram showed a severe blockage in my artery and they put a stent in my leg all the way up to my thigh in hopes of opening up the blockage. I was told I not only was going to lose my toe, but my entire leg would need to be amputated.

Not willing to accept such a severe diagnosis, I asked for a second opinion and was taken by ambulance to UMHS, trying not to move and putting constant pressure on my leg where I was told. Once again, the amazing doctors at UMHS gave me hope. Bypass surgery on my foot was scheduled for October 31, 1997. The doctors were able to take a part of the artery in my ankle and put it into my foot to create the necessary blood flow. Not only was the surgery a success, but I still even had my big toe!

The skin on the top of my foot, however, was not faring so well. Three weeks after the bypass surgery, I had an infection called cellulitis on my foot. It had eaten away nearly all of the skin on the top of my foot. After a two-week hospital stay and skin grafting done in hopes of repairing the damage, my foot was saved from having to be amputated. I lucked out yet again. Thanks to the amazing doctors and staff at the UMHS, I am proud to say I still have my right foot.

I had to be out of work for approximately eighteen months due to the surgery on my foot, and when I did finally go back to work, I had to use a walking cast for roughly five years. There were a couple of good years after that until the fifth metatarsal in my right foot decided to break unexpectedly. Unfortunately, this is the kind of thing that can happen when your body has been put through stress and multiple medications. I ended up with a walking cast again for another five years. Although my health was not perfect throughout those years, I was incredibly grateful for each day, to be able to experience life, and to have my freedom—away from being hooked up to a machine for several hours each week. I continued to work, exercise, and watch my diet daily. I vowed to never take my health for granted as I may have done occasionally in my earlier years.

In 2007 I went in for routine testing and the labs and numbers were not good. The antirejection medication I had been on for many years had started to become toxic to my kidney, and I was immediately put back on dialysis three days per week at a UMHS clinic. This time my body was more accepting of the hemodialysis, and a port was inserted into my neck. A fistula was put in place making my bicep look like a camel's back, but who was I to complain? I still had my life and hope for the future, as I always have. I would usually do the 5 a.m. shift and walk in the room with a cheerful smile. I would do my best to make the patients and nurses laugh before getting some much needed sleep while on the machine. I was on the transplant list in Ohio and Michigan and was hopeful I would qualify again if the stars were aligned a certain way.

I ended up joining a six-person swap to try and help others while, hopefully, helping myself obtain a new kidney. We were waiting on one more person with a certain blood type to join in order to make it all happen. During that time, I received a call for a kidney from Ohio and decided to turn it down because I felt obligated to the others in my swap team and did not want to let them down. I have always believed in putting others before me, and in that moment, it just seemed like the right thing to do. As they say, however, hindsight is always 20/20.

Two weeks after turning down that kidney, someone within the swap failed the health test and the entire plan fell apart. My doctor told me to never do something like that again, and all I could do at the time was laugh, because even though I understood why, I had to follow my heart at the time. At least I knew some other person in need received the kidney I gave up that day. I remained positive because I knew something was in store for me, and God had a plan.

I was celebrating my close friend's son's birthday with people I have known for most of my life. I had no idea how my life would change that day, and anytime I reflect upon it, I am utterly overwhelmed by the moment I heard the words from the woman I now refer to as my angel. Her name is Carrie. She is the wife of one of my closest childhood friends, Mark. Carrie and Mark were dating at the time and although I knew her to be a wonderful person who made a great friend of mine very happy, I had no idea she was an actual, living, breathing angel walking this earth. I will never forget the moment she asked me what blood type I was; I said B positive. She replied that was hers as well, and without hesitation, she offered to give me one of her kidneys.

I was stunned. I remember initially laughing it off and telling her how kind of her to say such a thing, but also unnecessary. I assured her I would be fine and she need not worry. Carrie, however, was not worried at all. In fact, she never showed an ounce of hesitation or fear and immediately insisted I give her the number for where she needed to call. When she told me she did not receive a return call, she asked me to make a call. So I did. They sent out the tubes for us both to have our blood drawn. We did as we were told and sent them back on December 5, 2010. We waited.

It was around the second week of January, 2011. I was driving home from dialysis, which was a huge part of my life at the time. I had spent the better part of my 40s driving to and from dialysis, spending approximately four hours per day, three days a week, in a chair hooked up to the machine required to cleanse and detoxify my body. It was not fun, although I always tried to make the most of it. While I was driving, Carrie called and exclaimed that we were a match! I remember having to pull over because tears filled my eyes when the words came out of her mouth and through the phone. I could hardly believe this amazing person—this angel—who hardly knew me at the time was willing to give me the most incredible gift of freedom from the chain of dialysis and a chance at having my life back.

Carrie never wanted recognition or praise, although I made sure to let all our family and friends know. She and I even ended up in the local newspaper after all was said and done, despite her efforts to remain unrecognized and under the radar. I just couldn't let that happen, as I was completely in awe of her selflessness and generosity. To this day, I always try to celebrate the anniversary of our surgeries: May 19, 2011, the day after my 45th birthday. I am forever grateful to Carrie for giving me the gift of another chance at life. After being on dialysis for almost five years prior to receiving her kidney, Carrie gave me the gift of freedom from dialysis.

Many people do not understand what being on dialysis entails. It not only requires a significant amount of your time each week, but there is also a grueling, specific diet that must be adhered to; otherwise, the body will pay for it, and the cleansing process will take much longer. The doctors also strongly suggest keeping in good physical shape while being on dialysis, which requires even more time. I would always show up with a smile on my face and try to leave on a positive note, but the truth is that dialysis basically became my life. I would miss out on certain special and meaningful events because of it. Making time for loved ones and attempting to form new relationships with others became somewhat of a chore at times. Dialysis, along with working full-time (and sometimes mandatory overtime), exercising regularly, constantly watching my diet, and trying to maintain a household and complete normal everyday chores left me exhausted. Being on dialysis also created problems for me in relation to my bladder. I had to intake a certain amount of water to help avoid blood clots that would form due to my pancreas and bladder being connected in my initial transplant surgery. On dialysis, I had to refrain from water to a certain extent and blood clots formed like kidney stones in my bladder. At one point, urination was impossible, and I had to be catheterized in order to break it up. I am not one to complain often about pain but I will say that it is hard to comprehend just how painful something like that can be if a person has not gone through it. Suffice to say, I am not a huge fan of dialysis, although I am, of course, grateful it is an option for people in need.

There have been a few setbacks with my most recent kidney transplant from Carrie, as there usually are. I had to have a peritoneal window surgery performed when my leg started experiencing extreme swelling from fluids due to the lymphedema caused by my transplant surgery. Thankfully, that surgery was a success and fluids began to drain normally once again. I had a severe bowel obstruction, which caused me to vomit profusely all the way to the hospital. After receiving an uncomfortable enema and strong medication, I finally had a bowel movement. Shortly thereafter, I was made aware that several hernias had formed within my abdomen and needed to be repaired. I spent roughly a month and a half in the hospital after that surgery and finally went back to work after three months.

In May 2012, I noticed a lump on the top of my head that turned out to be squamous cell cancer, caused by some of the medications I was taking, combined with not wearing a hat in the sun. My skin is more susceptible to cancer because of the antirejection medication I am on, which also suppresses my immune system. I had the lump removed that afternoon, immediately bought a hat, and took my great niece to the fair, as promised. I have always tried very hard to not let the setbacks bring me down and interfere with my enjoyment of life.

Being on dialysis for multiple years has taken quite a toll on my circulatory system. In December 2014, I was scheduled for a left leg arterial bypass and to have my left big toe amputated. Everything went as well as possible, and after one day of physical therapy, I was up on my leg. I was back to work within four months. The most unfortunate part about that is I can no longer wear flip-flops.

The biggest setback this past year has been the cellulitis that made a comeback. It switched over to the right foot from an infection on the toe. The blood infection caused my pancreas to slow down and, unfortunately, I am back on insulin. My donor kidney from Carrie still seems to be working well. I was able to return to work sometime in March 2017, thankfully, due to the work from the great doctors and staff at UMHS.

Life has its ups and downs. It is a roller coaster of problems and solutions, peaks and valleys. Some of the most common and usual freedoms are taken for granted. Many people assume life has a beginning and an end, and no matter the challenges or amount of time in between, we all will experience death one day. It seems so simple. We're all given a life to enjoy and live to the fullest until the end.

For me, life has not always been so simple. Most young people have adventurous experiences and don't think twice about not waking up the next morning or not being able to see again. I was not able to be so carefree. Between the illnesses that consumed much of my life and being on the verge of death twice before I had even reached the age of 50, I like to think I have an entirely different perspective than most. Because of this perspective and after many years dealing with health issues—being in and out of hospitals and on and off of dialysis—I decided to become a kidney transplant mentor for UMHS as a way of paying it forward.

Although my life is not what I expected, and I have been through more than most could imagine, I also have to say I am grateful it was me and not a loved one or anyone else going through it. I feel the pain, negativity, and struggles have made an unforgettable impact on not only me, but my friends, family, and even strangers. The difficulties in my life have shown me and those who surround me just how amazing life really is. Most think they are having a terrible day when they don't get enough sleep or if they are stressed about something. That was me at one point in my life, also. However, my experiences have shown me how amazing life is when health problems don't get in the way. I no longer complain about simple problems. Instead, I laugh and enjoy the small issues life has offered me.

All of the positivity I had during my medical problems didn't just come naturally to me. Others motivated me to take a risk, to break from the problems and take a shot at being free. I am lucky enough to have met so many wonderful people along my journey. As I face the next chapters in my life, I look forward to the many new friendships and experiences to come. The staff at UMHS made this positive environment for me that encouraged me to move forward with the transplants. I appreciate them for this every single day. I will continue to hold my head high throughout the future and whatever comes my way because I have been given the gift of freedom, the gift of life, and at the end of the day, I have been blessed.

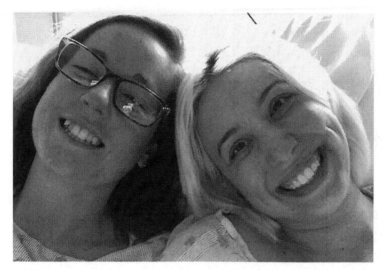

Shannon (left) and Lisa (right)

# Shannon's Story

Shannon was diagnosed with polycystic kidney disease and received a transplant at 32 years old from a living donor.

Learning you will one day need to have a kidney transplant is something a young child isn't prepared to understand. But that was me as a 12 year old being diagnosed with a genetic kidney disease. Going through this journey made me the person I am today. I don't think I would be this strong if I had not endured this experience. Some people ask me how I do it. I just say, "I don't know. You just pick up the pieces and keep on going." It's what needs to be done. Here is the story of the dying girl who was brought back to life one day in the drive-through of a Taco Bell.

As a young lady, you should be worried about school, boys, and what to wear the next day so you and your best friend don't match. But what do you do when that isn't the only thing you have to worry about? My father was diagnosed with polycystic kidney disease (PKD) in his mid-twenties. When he started to have health problems, both my parents wondered what to do. They learned that this illness could be passed down to their children. My mom now says that if she knew he had this disease, she might not have had us. That was hard to hear because no matter what happened to my premature child, I wouldn't have changed that for the world. But we will get into that later.

After learning both my brother and I could have this disease, we were tested. We had an ultrasound and, as suspected, both my brother and I carried the disorder. But only mine became active during puberty.

As a kid, you keep living, not knowing what the future brings and the hardship this diagnosis would have on you. I still played sports and was in band, and I had a 3.87 grade point average at graduation. I met and fell in love with my high school sweetheart who later would become my husband, but let's not get ahead of ourselves.

It was just before I turned 19 when the symptoms started. I still didn't think much of it and continued to live my life. All I had at that point was high blood pressure. I thought, "Heck, if I control it, we should be fine." You never know how sick you are until you're not sick anymore. Looking back, I had a lot of signs way before I knew how sick I was.

Like I said, I continued my life. My sweetheart and I got married, and then we decided to have a child. We were young, and there was no reason not to—so we thought. My primary doctor never really got my blood pressure under control, and I wasn't seeing a nephrologist at that point. So naturally, the doctor thought I was a typical case and took me on as a pregnant woman. It was only during the pregnancy that things started to go downhill. My blood pressure kept climbing, and I was becoming anemic. My body didn't know what to do, so it went into survival mode, and that's when it all went wrong.

I was hospitalized at 23 weeks of pregnancy with a blood pressure of 210/120 (normal is 120/80). I had preeclampsia and was about to have a seizure or stroke. During the few days before they took my child via C-section, my kidneys shut down. This was a real concern because in their poor state they may not have restarted. My platelets dropped to an alarming number, so the doctors waited until they went up, and then one morning the doctor came into my room and said they were taking the baby within the hour. I was instructed to call whomever I needed, and then the physician walked back out. The feeling you have at that point is without words. My daughter was born at only 15 ounces and

10 ½ inches long. My body didn't want to reboot, per se, until one night my stats went sky high and then crashed. I was in and out of consciousness for days.

The real symptoms started after that. I began to have episodes of pain and swollen kidneys which required a high level of narcotics. Over the next few years, my abdominal area enlarged, and it became harder to breathe and eat. In 2012, the pain had gotten so bad that my doctor considered having one of my kidneys removed to make more room. That was when he sent a referral to a hospital that wouldn't see me yet because I wasn't sick enough to be a patient. I was then referred to University of Michigan Health System (UMHS). By this point in my life, our daughter was old enough that she wasn't going to doctors all the time, and I could take a step back to focus on my health. I couldn't breathe, I barely ate, I felt sick all the time, and I would sleep most of the day. If I wasn't working or caring for my family, I was sleeping.

Let me tell you, I was freezing cold all the time. In the summer, if it was 70 degrees, sunny, and no breeze, I was in pants and a long-sleeve shirt. This was hard for me because I was used to being on the go without stopping. To not be able to do the things I loved was awful. Once I met with the doctor at UMHS, he wanted to do a procedure to help with the limited space in my stomach. He went in and popped my cysts and damaged them so they wouldn't grow back in that spot. This helped a bit, but it did have side effects as well. It dropped my glomerular filtration rate (GFR) to 20 percent, which allowed me to go on the kidney transplant list.

That was when I started looking for a kidney donor. The first candidate was my cousin. She was a match, but when it came time to launch the process, her husband said, "No." This was a huge blow to my emotional state. I stopped talking about it and went about my life as if it were normal. Then, I had an angel at work who started the process, and who, once again, was found to be a match. Unfortunately, her family was not on board.

Now, I know what you are thinking: how did you get so lucky to have two matches? I'm not sure—only God knows. During all the disappointment, we, as a family, decided not to share any more about it until we had a match and the donation was definitely going to happen.

As I worked, day in and day out, I started showing more signs of decline. I could not do things as fast as I used to; I was tired all the time and very short-fused. I kept my head up high and did what needed to be done. Work was getting harder to do, and one girl seemed to be fascinated with me and my disease. She started asking me questions all the time but was worried it bothered me. It didn't, so I answered all that I could. Then one day she wondered, "How does someone go about getting tested to help?" I gave her the information and went about my day. A few weeks later, I got another packet in the mail to give blood for a potential donor. I went and did it, like before, but didn't get my hopes up. This poor girl kept on asking me if I wanted her to do it, and sadly, I was unable to answer her, which made her frustrated. I just kept saying, "You must make that decision on your own. If I give you an answer, that may sway your decision."

As luck would have it, God worked in her and told her she needed to do this. On that fateful day at Taco Bell, she called and said she had scheduled our surgery for March 5, 2014. The whole family was beyond excited. No words could ever come close to describing what she had done for this family. Thankfully, I could avoid dialysis and a long wait on the list. Unfortunately, I did have to have an arteriovenous (AV) fistula placed to prepare for dialysis. Many people have asked me how I stayed so upbeat. The only thing I can tell you is that I believe in God, and He has always comforted me. I was never afraid of dying, and if that was what had to happen, then that was His choice, not mine.

Over the next few months, my donor and I got to know each other better and our families got to spend time together. My donor didn't want recognition for doing this; she did it because it was the right thing to do. She was funny: she didn't want to tell anyone at work. I laughed and said, "What do you think they are going to think when we both leave at the same time and come back at the same time? What will you say happened to you?"

After the surgery, I felt much better—it was like night and day. I love to eat now and enjoy life so much more. I am able to do things again that used to be hard, and I am able to try new things. I have gone on motorcycle rides with my husband across the country and went to Disneyland with my daughter. Before, I was unable to stay awake or move enough to do that stuff. There are still days where my old kidneys act up and hurt, but I know they will run their course and one day I won't have to deal with that.

After the transplant, I have changed the way I do some things. I only drink pop occasionally, and I limit the protein I eat so I don't put extra strain on the new kidney. Drinking has stopped, even though I wasn't much of a drinker. I try to stay healthy, to do what the doctors say, and I never miss a medication. I set the alarm on my phone for twice a day to ensure I don't forget because we all know that when you are busy things can slip. My new kidney didn't grow on a tree, and I can't just get another one, so I take care of it.

If you know someone or are considering donating a kidney, please do. The pain is worth it, surgery is short, and recovery isn't long, but it can change a family's life forever. My husband and daughter were looking at losing their wife and mother but because one young woman gave up eight weeks of her life, I can now live. She is completely back to normal and since has had a healthy child; her pregnancy went perfectly. She has no long-term effects from any of this, just four stab-hole-size scars and one that is about four inches long where they removed the kidney. It is all laparoscopic nowadays.

Anyone and everyone who sees patients like this should think before making a judgment. You have no idea how these patients live or what they are going through. Take your time and listen to them. Sometimes, that is all people need.

Looking back on everything I went through from my teenage years, I feel that my experiences have made me a stronger person. I have always believed everything happens for a reason. I don't question it—I just go with it. God has a plan for you and your health: embrace it. Having my kidney transplant has helped me to not take anything for granted and to enjoy every day to the fullest.

Never forget to stop and smell the fresh air. I'm a happier person now and feel fantastic every day. The biggest challenge I had was me and not allowing myself to take in all that was happening. I was scared and didn't want to face my end, so I didn't. Now I see my future as bright and uplifting and, one day, I hope to help others who are in the same shoes as me. I hope my story helps you through a tough time.

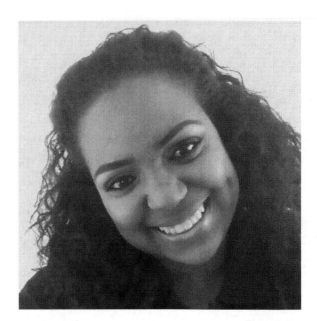

Taneisha

# Taneisha's Story

Taneisha was diagnosed with nephrotic syndrome and received a transplant at 25 years old from a living donor.

On September 21, 1990, I was diagnosed with nephrotic syndrome at the young age of eight. My family instantly began making lifestyle changes. We changed our eating and exercising habits. My family treated me just like any other child in the family. They spoiled me rotten. My cheeks grew chubby from the medications I took daily. I learned how to play violin, acoustic bass, swim, and even went on annual family trips to Myrtle Beach, Maryland, and sometimes Florida.

For the next 16 years, I lived the life any healthy human being would. I graduated from high school and attended an Ivy League Historically Black College and University (HBCU) fourteen hours away from home. I met amazing people and traveled with college buddies often. I did things some only dreamed about. I was having the time of my life.

In July 2006, I decided to go to Charlotte, North Carolina, with my cousin and best friend who had just accepted a job there. I was suddenly struck with fatigue and headaches. After driving myself to the hospital, I was diagnosed with end-stage renal disease (ESRD). This meant my kidneys had completely shut down. I started dialysis immediately. It never once registered that my life was in danger. I called my mom in Detroit, Michigan, who became my biggest advocate. My family drove down to Alabama to pack up my apartment and then drove to Charlotte to pick up my car and finally back to Detroit.

Once I arrived home, I moved in with my grandparents and started a new life—a life that included two nonfunctioning kidneys. For the next 18 months, I was on dialysis three times a week for four hours. My life was on pause, or so we thought. It was at this point that I learned the true meaning of strength. I became a fighter I never knew existed. My dialysis technician in North Carolina taught me the proper procedures for my care. She taught me that my dialysis catheter was my lifeline. It was to be taken seriously at all times. This catheter was placed in my superior vena cava where it stayed until transplant.

Yes, I said transplant. Without my knowledge, my courageous cousin, Krystal, had previously begun testing to become my living donor. With much prayer and meditation, she completed all of her testing and a transplant date was set. Krystal flew in from Maryland to donate one of her well-functioning kidneys to me. In the days leading up to the transplant, we had kidney parties, fish fries, and a family prayer service at church. We did television interviews and recorded a few health videos. We were destined for greatness! God was pointing us in directions we didn't know existed. On February 15, 2008, our lives changed for the better. Our transplant was a success. All of our family came together to celebrate such a miraculous occasion.

The morning of the surgery was like most other mornings. We were filled with hope, love, faith, trust, and compassion. We walked into that hospital as two and left as one. Our family gathered in the waiting room and formed a prayer circle. Then they individually came by to give their well wishes before we entered the operating room. They rolled Krystal off to surgery first and let me know I would be going in shortly after her. You could see the tears rolling down the cheeks of our family. You could see the hope glistening in their eyes. You could feel God's arms of protection all around us. It was finally my turn.

I woke up without knowledge of ever having been asleep. I needed to use the restroom. I kept telling this strange lady who was watching me that I needed to use the restroom. But for some odd reason, she kept telling me to go ahead and use it right there. I just couldn't believe this lady wanted me to wet myself. So I politely said, "Excuse me ma'am, but I am a grown woman and I cannot pee on myself."

This is when I heard the best news I could have heard. "You have a catheter in from your transplant." Now, most wouldn't think of that as being great news, but did you hear her say transplant? I had my transplant! I was so confused for a moment. Then the tears started flowing. All I wanted was my cousin. I couldn't believe I had a transplant and didn't know.

Well, I cried and cried and cried and cried. And cried some more. All I wanted to do was see my cousin. Finally, after all the crying, we were reunited. And guess what? She was crying, too. These were tears of appreciation and joy. Our family rejoiced in the waiting room after pacing the floor for four hours. Our parents hugged each other and cried together. It was such a joyous occasion.

During the recovery period in the hospital, our family showed up by the dozens. Every day the family room was filled with a minimum of 25 people. They took turns running between the two rooms. We had and still have the best support system. I remember telling my aunt, "I am peeing now." She was so overjoyed. For years after the transplant, she would often ask me, with a grin on her face, if I was still peeing. It is often the simple things we take for granted.

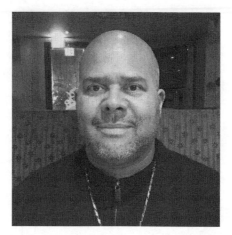

Tyrone

# Tyrone's Story

Tyrone was diagnosed with type 2 diabetes and received a transplant at 46 years old from a deceased donor.

I would like to start off by acknowledging all those who motivated, supported, and inspired me during my battle with kidney disease. The list includes my wife, kids, parents, brothers, family, friends, and healthcare professionals. My battle with kidney disease will hopefully encourage others to realize that life should be lived and not ended.

I believe my kidney disease began when I started working the midnight shift as a patient equipment attendant at the hospital. I have worked there for over 25 years. I worked the afternoon shift in the beginning of my career, and my wife commuted to her job in Detroit every day. We have two children, and at that time, our older son was in kindergarten and our younger son was only a baby. So as a compromise to daycare, I decided to work the midnight shift. I have been working this shift for 22 years now. Due to a lack of sleep, not eating right, and a family history of diabetes and high blood pressure, I developed my kidney disease.

When I was first diagnosed with high blood pressure, it was controllable. However, instead of the doctor advising me to eat right and try to lose weight on my own, he just put me on a pill right away. Now I am not saying the medication increased my blood pressure, but it certainly was something that I felt sealed my fate. In my mind, once you start taking medication to control any health issue, it is very hard to ease off of it. This caused anger at first, and I felt I should have spoken up more about my health. Don't just assume the first diagnosis is the best one. I should have asked more questions.

Then, after about five years of working the midnight shift with my blood pressure continually rising, I developed diabetes. This is how the journey began that led me to kidney disease. By having a combination of these two deadly illnesses, I pretty much felt this sealed my fate. My nephrologist told me my kidneys were functioning at 25 percent and this would eventually lead to dialysis. About two weeks later I received a fistula to prepare me. However, this didn't lead to me taking better care of myself. I am one who enjoys life, and a part of that enjoyment was traveling, eating great food, and enjoying family. This enjoyment eventually caught up with me when, one day, I started gaining weight. It all seemed to happen suddenly. It seemed like every day I was gaining about ten pounds. It was hard for me to breathe and walk. I knew deep down what was happening to me, but I was in denial. The weight gain was actually fluid building up in my body. I feared I would be on dialysis for the rest of my life.

The conversation about my high blood pressure and diabetes was relayed to family and friends. However, the seriousness of my kidney disease was only shared with my wife at the time. When I started gaining weight, I started getting attention from my family and friends. They forced me to go to the hospital, and this is when reality set in. The doctor on duty told me I had to start dialysis right away. I was told I had bad blood and my kidneys weren't functioning properly. This trip to the Emergency Room ended up with me being put on dialysis for three days a week, four hours each day, for four years.

I felt like this was a death sentence because I knew my normal lifestyle would change dramatically. I wouldn't be able to travel the way I wanted. I wouldn't be able to be at family events. Even thoughts about me working a normal shift would be affected. I started thinking about no longer being here with my family and friends. I wanted to pray, but I was questioning God about why I was chosen to have this disease. I started preparing for death by creating a bucket list and making sure my family would be taken care of with insurance plans.

While on dialysis, the doctors were telling me that my chances would be better if I was placed on a waitlist for a kidney transplant than to remain on dialysis for the rest of my life. I still struggled with this decision because I didn't want to be on a waitlist for a kidney. At the same time, I remained optimistic that I would be able to enjoy a normal life. I also had to make a decision about receiving a kidney from a living or deceased donor. After talking to my younger brother, he said he would be a donor for me. Unfortunately, even though he has the same blood type, he also had high blood pressure so he wasn't allowed to give me his kidney. My wife, seeing me in anguish and pain, stepped in to be a donor for me. I did not want her or my brother to do this, even though it was the ultimate sacrifice they would be making for me. I just couldn't allow my wife to make the decision to do this for me.

I kept my spirits up by living my life. I worked double shifts at the hospital, increased my exercise, traveled within my dialysis time frame, enjoyed concerts, and took care of my ailing parents. People (including doctors and other healthcare professionals) considered me an example and a miracle that I was able to do all these things and still be on dialysis. I never allowed myself to show that I was mentally, physically, or emotionally exhausted. I wanted to be strong for everyone else.

I remember when I received that lifesaving phone call from the hospital that a kidney had been found for me. There were some traumatic events happening in my family at the same time. My wife's parents had both been diagnosed with lung cancer. Her mother had to have immediate surgery to remove part of her lung (she is now in remission). My wife's father did not survive. We were heading to Nashville, Tennessee, to see him when I received the phone call about my kidney. I was very torn and had mixed feelings. I had to make the decision to turn around to go to the hospital. My wife and her brother would not be able to see their father for the last time. However, they were very supportive and happy to hear I would receive this kidney. They were at the hospital throughout the whole process.

After my kidney transplant, I changed my eating habits, exercised more, kept in touch with my doctors, made my appointments, stuck to my medication schedule, and made sure to keep up with blood draws. My advice to others is to stay mentally and physically healthy when it comes time to consider a kidney transplant. Physically, maintain a healthy weight. Mentally, keep a positive attitude and seek the support of family and friends to help you. I am able to travel longer now than just a weekend and able to attend more family functions. I felt like I was in prison and locked down before my kidney transplant. Now I feel more free to enjoy my life.

I know that life is not promised, but it is to be enjoyed each and every day that you are here. I am now taking advantage of that. I am enjoying time with my granddaughter, and I have traveled to places I dreamed about—like Puerto Rico and Niagara Falls. I am able to be a much stronger person after being challenged with this disease that I could have died from.

I thank my family, my friends, my healthcare team, and coworkers for their support.

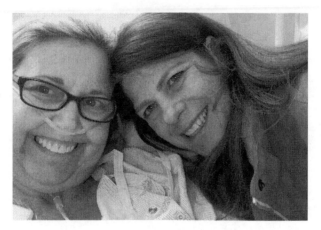

Crystal (left) and Maria (right)

# Crystal's Story

Crystal was diagnosed with membranoproliferative glomerulonephritis (MPGN) and received transplants at 24, 35, and 49 years old. The first transplant was from a deceased donor; the second and third transplants were from living donors.

W here to begin? My story is a long one, and it includes three transplants. It started with an allergic reaction to kittens when I was eight years old. In 1976, I was visiting my dad in Hawaii where he was stationed as an Army officer. He rushed me to the Army hospital because my eyes were swollen, and I had welts on my wrists and stomach. I had played with kittens before but had not had a reaction like this. The Emergency Room staff determined I was having an allergic reaction, but they also ran some generic tests for blood and urine to ensure nothing else was going on. The results from the tests showed I had blood and protein in my urine and complements of protein in my blood. I don't recall the exact abnormalities with my blood work, but as a result, they admitted me to the hospital.

Purely by coincidence, the doctor assigned to my case had just been to a kidney conference and realized that my blood and urine results were indicative of a kidney disorder. The doctor got me stabilized in a couple of days and allowed me to return home.

At that time, I was so young I did not understand the full impact of what was wrong with me. The doctors did not know the full impact either. Kidney diagnoses were not as prevalent then as they are today. I continued to have regular doctor visits for the next few years until I had a kidney biopsy when I was 12 years old; I remember it hurt terribly.

I was lying down on my stomach with a pillow under my belly to push my kidneys toward the top of my back. This made it easier for the doctor to insert a large needle into my kidney to grab a piece for analysis. They used an ultrasound machine to pinpoint the location of the kidney and how deep the kidney was from the surface. They marked the location and numbed the area. Then, they inserted the special, long needle into the kidney and grabbed a very small piece. The numbing helped the pain, but I did feel the pressure. I remember I had to stay home from school for about a week, as it was hard for me to carry all my books to school.

The biopsy came back with a diagnosis of membranoproliferative glomerulonephritis, now called MPGN. The disease was thickening the membranes of the kidney until the kidney could no longer filter. When this happened, I would need a kidney transplant.

The doctors put me on high doses of IV steroids to try to knock the problem away. I was admitted to the hospital over the Christmas holiday so I did not miss any more school. I remember people coming around, bringing us gifts and crafts. I was in the hospital for about a week and was then sent home. It took time to see if the steroids were going to reverse the kidney problem. When this did not happen, they started to taper me off.

The steroids caused me to be ravenous, and I gained 30 pounds on my 87-pound frame. I had huge chipmunk cheeks, a huge belly, extra fat at the top of my back like a dowager's hump, and extra hair all over. In those days, people did not come into the classroom to explain why some kids may be different because they were encountering medical issues. As a result, the kids teased me terribly, and I felt excluded. The kids thought there was something really wrong with me. The worst memory I had was a girl calling me, "Miss Piggy." With these experiences, I swore I would never go on prednisone/steroids ever again. I did not want to go through the body changes and mood swings that are a symptom of steroids.

The high doses of steroids did not change the status of my kidney disease. From age 12 until I finished college, my doctors monitored my progress. I would go to the doctor twice a year. If something changed, they would shorten the amount of time between visits. While I was in college, I started noticing extra fluid on my ankles. After one of my doctor visits, the doctor prescribed diuretics to remove the extra water off my legs. I dropped 12 pounds and my friends were jealous.

Luckily for me, I was able to enjoy a full college life. I was part of a sorority and made friendships that I still have today. My disease was impacting the things I could handle or participate in, but only a little bit. I was able to do what everyone else was doing, just not to the same extent as everyone else. I was fortunate enough not to feel that I had missed anything.

I was in complete denial that I would need a kidney transplant, even though I had been told it was inevitable since I was a child. Sometime in 1990, my doctor noticed my lab results were changing. I got to work one Monday and had a horrible headache, and I could not stop throwing up. I was 22 years old and was still going out with friends to drink. I had been out the previous weekend so I thought I was sick due to a hangover and chalked it up to that.

The next Monday, I got sick again, and I had not been out that week nor on the weekend. I knew there had to be something wrong. My internal medicine doctor was working with my nephrologist. My blood pressure had been climbing lately. One of the medications they prescribed could cause rebound hypertension, which could cause my blood pressure to start climbing out of control. Knowing this, I called the internal medicine doctor and let her know what had been happening. She told me to get to her office immediately.

On the way to the doctor's office, I had to pull over many times to be sick, and I had another horrible headache. When I got there, my blood pressure was 220/160. My doctor was very concerned and sent me to the Emergency Room where I was admitted to the hospital. They got the nausea under control, but it took three days to get rid of the headache. They gave me medicine to bring down my blood pressure to a normal level. When my headache went away, they sent me home with new blood pressure medications. They mentioned that my kidney was starting not to work as well as it had been, and I would need to see the nephrologist more often. But I was still in denial that I would need a transplant.

I continued to go out with my friends, which was typically on Thursday, Friday, and Saturday evenings. Going out was mostly about dancing for me. I was moderating my alcohol content, keeping in mind that not being able to take my blood pressure medication had resulted in a trip to the Emergency Room.

I began seeing a new nephrology doctor. Based on the decline of my kidneys, he thought it would be best to create an access for dialysis. I was horrified. I was 23 years old, and the last thing I wanted was some surgery on my arm to prepare me for dialysis. Even worse, the doctor wanted to put it in my left arm where everyone would see it. I left the office in tears, determined that I did not need this yet. When I went back for my second appointment, I was met with the same decision to make. Again, I was in tears and decided I needed another doctor who understood me better and did not make me cry every time I left his office.

My new doctor allowed my kidney to deteriorate without having a prior surgery to create a fistula. He also agreed to let me put the fistula in my upper left arm, which made it less obvious to others. He had the right attitude for me. He let me live my life while I could and would handle the failure when it occurred.

As I got sicker, I could only go out with my friends on Fridays and Saturdays because I could sleep in on Saturday and Sunday mornings. This lasted for a while until I could only go out on Saturday. I was starting not to feel well. I had a bad taste in my mouth, was overly tired, and I did not feel like eating. I was starting to lose weight and it was harder for me to do anything. I needed more and more sleep as I got sicker. I was seeing my nephrologist on a regular basis with the amount of time between visits getting shorter. My doctor basically let me go on doing what I could until I could not do anything anymore. He knew when I wasn't going out any longer that I was close to kidney failure. I eventually got so sick I ended up at the Emergency Room and was admitted again.

They put a catheter in my chest for me to get dialysis. They got me stabilized and on dialysis three times a week. Then, they set up surgery to create a fistula for me.

My chest catheter had two lines connected to my artery. One of the lines was an arterial access and the other was a venous access. The arterial line took the blood out of my body and sent it to the dialysis machine to clean my blood. The clean blood was then put back into my body via the venous access. This process took two- to three-and-one-half hours. At that point I was still working full-time and working toward my master's degree. When I got really sick, I sometimes had to delay taking classes.

Both work and class kept me from thinking too much about what I was going through. The actual reality was that I was in kidney failure and would remain on dialysis unless I got a kidney transplant. In 1991, kidney transplants were still new in the medical world. I was at a hospital in Washington, D.C., and their transplant waitlist was about a year long. Transplants from living donors were not a common occurrence and were only allowed from family members. I had a small family—one sister, a mom, and a dad. My sister was tested, and she was not a match for me. My mom was ruled out for health reasons. My dad decided it was not something he could do at that time, as he had to support his family. I had no one to donate for me, so I waited on the list.

In June 1992, I got the call. In those days, cell phones were not widely used, and I was given a pager to reach me when a kidney became available. I had let the battery die on the pager, but my husband was reachable and he knew how to reach me. He called around my office and my boss answered the phone. She came running down the hall to our conference room and let me know that they had a kidney. I needed to get to the hospital as soon as possible.

This was the first time I had been called for a kidney. There were a number of things that could happen. We were told you may not receive a kidney when called if the cross-match was positive, you were sick, or the kidney had an issue. I headed to the hospital confident that this was the kidney for me. I had faith and knew my situation was in God's hands. If this kidney was meant for me, it would happen. If not, another one would become available.

The tests were run and the cross-match was negative. The kidney was in perfect shape except the artery had been cut a little short. And, I was healthy. We were a go for the transplant.

The transplant was scheduled to begin early the next morning. The kidney arrived from Philadelphia. It was packed on ice in a Styrofoam cooler marked "Fragile" and "Transplant Organ." I wasn't able to see inside, but I was able to pat it and tell it to be good for me. I made a silent prayer for success with the surgery. I had to take a shower on the morning of the transplant and wash my entire body with red cleanser to stop the spread of any germs that may have collected on my body. I went to surgery with my hair wet.

I had been told the surgery would be quick, about 30 minutes. My family became concerned when I was not out of surgery after three hours. They were told the surgery was taking longer because the kidney's artery needed to be extended. Once it was connected, I immediately started to feel the urge to urinate. My kidney produced urine from the start. I woke up telling the staff, "I have to pee!" A catheter was inserted to manage my urine output.

I was attached to all sorts of IV bags to keep my kidney working and flushing fluids. My new kidney was working like a champ. Back then, they were still working out the kinks with transplants. I was put on immunosuppressant medications, starting on larger doses which were then tapered down to a manageable level.

I had many setbacks with my first transplant and was in and out of the hospital for five months. I had two episodes of rejection that required heavy-duty IV immunosuppressant drugs over a period of time, and the kidney was saved. Then I got cytomegalovirus (CMV). I had not been exposed to CMV, but the kidney had. I was on antiviral IV medication for two weeks and was pretty sick, but we got through this.

I then started to become very anemic. My hemoglobin and hematocrit were decreasing rather rapidly. While on dialysis, the dialysis clinic typically gives a synthetic version of a hormone three times a week. When you get a transplant, you do not need this medication any longer as your new kidney takes over and creates it for you. In my case, this was not happening.

They stopped two of the medications thinking one of these might be causing the deterioration. I started taking the synthetic hormone again, and I have been on this medication ever since. They were not sure I was going to survive this severe anemia. My hematocrit had dropped to 14 and was continuing to drop. I was admitted to the hospital and given two pints of blood.

This was not long after the HIV virus had become known to the public. From that time forward, when I needed blood, I was very concerned I was going to get HIV so I would try to avoid getting blood transfusions. I was admitted to the hospital many times after this transplant for urinary tract infections (UTIs). Since my urinary tract had been rerouted, the doctors were concerned that a UTI could progress and go to my kidney. To keep this from happening, they would admit me and give me IV antibiotics. I would not feel sick but would have to be in the hospital when this happened.

I got frustrated at being in the hospital so many times, but eventually I realized that was where I needed to be. I quit complaining, and I accepted it. I knew this would help me to keep my kidney.

After five months of different complications and being admitted to the hospital many times, my body stabilized, and life with my first kidney began. The amount of time between my doctor visits spread out until I was seeing the doctor every six months. I resumed working and slowly got back into my life again. I was so very thankful that I was no longer on dialysis and was living like all my other friends.

About nine years later, I started feeling not right and was having trouble with my blood pressure so I began seeing my nephrologist more frequently. First, every four months, then every two months. It was at one of these visits that they said I would need to get a kidney biopsy to see how my kidney was functioning. I was concerned, but I continued with my life until told otherwise.

I went to Myrtle Beach on vacation with girlfriends that August. It was frustrating for me as I was very tired and could not keep up with them. I stayed back from some activities so I could take a nap. I made the most of the trip, but knew my kidney was not keeping up.

When I got home from the trip, I had multiple voicemail messages from the transplant office urging me to call to schedule a biopsy. My recent lab results were not good; they required a biopsy to see if I was rejecting. If I was rejecting, it could be acute (meaning they could give me medication to stop the rejection) or chronic (meaning there was nothing they could do to save the kidney).

A biopsy on a transplant kidney is much easier than on your native kidneys. Because the transplant kidney is in the front pelvic region, the biopsy needle did not have to go far and was not as painful. I got the results of the biopsy the next week and, unfortunately, I was in chronic kidney failure. There was nothing the doctors could do to stop the rejection. When they told me the news, I was devastated and scared. I broke down in tears. The nurse was very understanding and let me voice my frustration and fears. I had been through kidney failure before, and I knew what was coming. I would start feeling crappy most of the time, would have to adjust my diet to a kidney-friendly diet (low protein, low phosphorus, low potassium, low salt, and low fat), and would eventually return to dialysis. I did not look forward to any of these changes. I had my biopsy in July 2001 and was told my kidney failure would most likely be coming quickly.

I stayed off dialysis until February of the next year. I had gone through the kidney transplant evaluation process at the University of Michigan (U-M) Transplant Center but knew I needed to find a kidney another way as the wait was four- to five-years long. I did not want to be on dialysis that long. I had other things to do with my life.

I started talking with family and friends about a kidney donation. For my first transplant, only family members were allowed to donate. Now, anyone could be a donor. My dad was going to donate for me this time. He went through the tests and evaluation process. All the testing had been going great, and he had one more test to complete. My dad called to tell me the results, and it was not what I was expecting.

"I have good news and bad news," he said.

"Give me the bad news first," I said.

He responded, "I can't donate a kidney for you." I was so surprised when he said this. My dad had been in the Army for 27 years and was very active and healthy.

"So what is the good news?" I said.

"You may have saved my life! They found I have an aneurysm on my aorta, and because of this test, they are aware of it so they can keep watching it. If they had not found it, it may have ruptured and killed me."

How do you respond to that? I told my dad I was glad they found the aneurysm, but I was crushed inside. Dialysis keeps you alive until you get a transplant, but it is no fun and very time consuming. My hope of avoiding dialysis was dwindling. I was determined to find a living donor. I knew that a transplant's longevity is better from a living donor compared to a kidney from the waiting list. I also knew I could only get so many kidneys in my lifetime. I wanted a living-donor kidney.

My sister was not willing to donate as she was concerned that one of her children would need a kidney one day. She had been tested when I needed the first transplant, but at that time they said I could get a better match from the waiting list. Now her children had a very small probability of contracting a kidney disease, plus the doctors would not allow her to donate because she was not healthy enough to do it. My family gene pool was exhausted.

During this time, my friends had been listening as I told them about the people who had been tested. My friends were sympathetic. One of them said she would get tested to see if she could donate for me. It turned out she was a match, so she started the testing process. She ended up passing all the tests, and we were ready to set a date for surgery.

My friend talked to her husband about potential dates for surgery, and he freaked out. He did not understand that the testing his wife had been doing was to prepare to give me a kidney, which would require her to be in the hospital and out of commission for four to six weeks (at the time, she was a stay-at-home wife with a three-year-old daughter). He said he didn't want her to donate. My friend reached out to her family, and they were also very concerned and didn't want her to do it. She reached out to her pastor for advice, and he also did not recommend that she donate since she had a young child to care for.

I distinctly remember her calling me, crying and apologizing that she could not donate for me. She really wanted to do this for me, but she did not have the support of her family, which is crucial. You would have expected she would have been consoling me, but I ended up consoling her. I know this is a hard decision for people to make. It is a harder surgery for the donor than for the recipient, and it takes longer to recuperate. In order for a person to donate, he or she needs to have the right mind-set and have faith that everything will be okay after the surgery. The person has to be positive. No hesitation.

After this, I knew it was going to be hard to find a donor. I had another girlfriend who was a single parent. She made an appointment for the evaluation. She also was not willing to donate after the evaluation. She realized it was difficult since she was a single parent and she would have to be off work for a period of time. I completely understood her position and was thankful she had considered it. I was disappointed though. Where was I going to find a donor?

To my surprise, my boyfriend decided to get tested. I was hoping he was serious about it and prayed he would be a match. He ended up matching me and passing all the tests. We were then ready to set a date for surgery. The date was set for Wednesday, October 2, 2002.

I remember that day like yesterday. My dad flew in to be with me for the surgery. My neighbor and two friends also came to the hospital before the surgery to support me. We were there when my boyfriend went back for his surgery. I talked to him before the surgery, and he was not himself. I had not seen him this way, but I didn't say anything. Everyone deals with stress differently. Afterward he told me that he had been afraid, but even with his fear, he still went through with it.

Many hours later, they took me back and gave me his kidney. It worked instantly, and I recall waking up feeling spasms in my bladder. The spasms were the result of the stent that was placed between the new kidney and the bladder. I woke up feeling better than I had felt in a long time and knew I would have my life back again. No more dialysis. I was free again and determined to keep this kidney even longer than the first one.

I was up walking the next day and out of the hospital by Friday. In those days, they had you come back on Saturday and Sunday, for six hours each day, for IV immunosuppressant drugs. Then you had to go back a week from Monday for labs, to see the doctor, and check how your kidney was doing.

After the doctor determined I was good to go, he asked me if I would mind talking to a family about my experience with the surgery. He had a patient whose sister was willing to donate but the patient was not willing to have the surgery as she was afraid it would hurt too much. She would rather end up on dialysis and forgo the transplant. I gladly agreed to talk with them.

The patient was there with her husband, her sister, and her sister's husband. I had my surgery one week prior to that day. I shared with them that this was my second transplant. I showed them my two surgical scars and they could see I was very mobile and not in serious pain. Don't get me wrong, it did hurt, but the pain medications made it very manageable. I really hoped that I was able to make an impression so the woman would let her sister donate and move forward with a transplant. I knew she would be much happier after that. My doctor said she did decide to go ahead with getting a transplant.

My second transplant was very uneventful. No rejection or additional hospital stays. I was back to work in five weeks and enjoying my life, free of dialysis. I am blessed to say that my second transplant lasted 14 years and two days.

I then had the biopsy that confirmed I was again in kidney failure in December 2014. But I was determined that I was going to do as much as I could before my kidney failed. In the two years it took for my kidney to get bad enough to need dialysis, I took my niece to Florida to visit my dad and to go to SeaWorld and Discovery Cove. I wanted to do things that someone would have on a bucket list. My husband and I went to Mexico for a week for some sun and fun. I loved the crystal blue water and white sand. I enjoyed it while I could, not knowing when we would be able to go on vacation again.

I had been sharing on Facebook that I was in kidney failure and looking for a living kidney donor. I had reconnected with two people I knew from high school over 30 years before. One of them contacted me and said he wanted to donate for me. I was so surprised by the offer and instantly brought to tears. Here was someone I had not seen or talked to in 30 years, but he was willing to donate a kidney for me. I was overwhelmed with emotion: hopeful, blessed, but cautious. I knew that finding a donor was not that simple. His heart was in the right place, but he was ruled out due to a chronic medical condition.

My last trip was to go back to Virginia for my 30-year high-school reunion and my 25-year college reunion. While there, I let people know I was in kidney failure and looking for a donor. If anyone expressed interest, I gave them the number for the Transplant Clinic so they could talk to a donor coordinator.

I knew at this point that the pool of people who would be willing to donate was very small. I also knew the wait for a kidney from a deceased donor was even longer than it had been 14 years before. Now the wait was five-to-seven years. I was determined not to wait that long. So, I started my mission to find a kidney.

I created a special Facebook page devoted to finding a living donor. I shared my story and updated it as my kidney failure progressed. I posted pictures and videos of my dialysis experience. My coworker created a sign to put on my car to get the word out even further. (It did not get too many responses.) Just getting the word out about kidney failure and its repercussions helps to better educate the public and to recruit living donors.

There have been about 50 people who have expressed interest in donating for me. The majority of them were ruled out for medical reasons. I found that, often, people in their late 40s to early 50s already have health issues that preclude them from donating. It is a challenge to find someone who is both willing and able to be a donor.

One day at work I was talking to my coworker, Maria. Somehow we began talking about how I needed a kidney transplant. I thought I had told her my story before, but apparently I had not. When I told it to her briefly, she looked at me and said, "I could do that." As many other people had said the same thing, I took it all in stride. She started the process of getting tested, and each time she passed the tests. Unfortunately, she was not a match for me so while she was willing to donate, her kidney would not help me. However, she was still willing to donate through the Paired Donation Program.

I received my third kidney transplant on March 1, 2017. My husband and I got up very early to be at the hospital by 5:30 a.m. I needed to be there early because I had to be cleared before my paired-donation donor went into surgery. I was cautiously optimistic that it was going to happen but didn't want to get my hopes up. The surgeons came by an hour or so later to let me know the donor was in the operating room and the procedure was happening. I was getting excited but still holding my heart back in case this did not happen.

When we checked in, the staff offered coloring books and crayons. I took some since I knew I would have plenty of time before my surgery. I was scheduled to start around noon. I had an IV in my arm but wasn't getting any fluid so I'm sure I was getting dehydrated. Since my kidney wasn't working very well, too much fluid would have been hard on my heart.

The surgeons passed by around noon and let me know that it was taking longer for the donor's surgery because they had to separate a lot of connective tissue from the kidney. The only thing I knew about my donor was that he was a male associated with Michigan Medicine.

Around 1 p.m. they were ready to take me to the operating room. I asked if they could wait to knock me out until after I got to the surgery room. We entered Operating Room 13. Many people would be anxious about this number, but over the years it had been a good number for me.

The surgery took five hours. I got to recovery at 6 p.m. When I finally woke up, I was burning up. They brought ice packs to put by my sides and behind my neck, plus a cold wash cloth on my face. They also found a small portable fan to blow on me. At 7 p.m. my husband, Gerry, could see me. He said I was red and puffy. He went home at 8 p.m. and his sister spent some time with me until about 9 p.m.

You would think having a transplant scheduled ahead of time would mean a room would be waiting for you. The floor I was on for kidney transplants was hopping. They would get one patient out and another one in within hours. I had to wait for one of these releases, especially since I had a private room. As an immune-compromised patient, I need as little contact with people as possible, especially sick people. I think I got to my room around 10:30 p.m. (I think I was sleeping until they got me there and then I probably slept some more.) I was given a pump to deliver pain medication for the first 24 hours, so I didn't feel much pain.

It was early Thursday morning, and I was being monitored closely by the staff. They came around-the-clock to take my vitals and make sure my kidney was working. They had put in a catheter during surgery so I would not have to get up to go to the bathroom. I had blood in my urine for four-to-five days, but it then started to go away.

They had started high doses of immunosuppressant medication by IV during surgery. When I got out of surgery and was hot and red, I learned I was having an allergic reaction to this medicine. We discovered this on the second day of receiving IV medicine. I noticed my forehead, my eyes, and my jaw were starting to itch. They gave me an antihistamine and some steroids, and many of the symptoms decreased. Then, the third time I needed the medicine, they gave me prophylactic medicines for the allergy. This time I was just fine with the IV infusion.

On Friday, Maria—my coworker and donor—had her surgery. I was able to see her after she got out. Once she got home, she started returning back to normal. The amazing thing is that she ran in a 10K event nine weeks later. She truly is an amazing and inspirational person, and I could never thank her enough for what she did.

I was released on Saturday and my husband took me home. My dad was arriving on Tuesday after my surgery. It turns out that was the afternoon of my first appointment after surgery. We had been told this would be a long appointment; I had many people to see and could expect it to take most of the day. Gerry and I made a plan; if he had to leave to get my dad, I would hang out and wait for him to return with my dad and we would all drive home together. Luckily, this didn't happen. We were able to get out of the clinic rather quickly with enough time to pick up my dad.

A couple days after this, I was feeling light-headed and had an increased heart rate. It felt like my heart was going to beat out of my chest. I tried to drink more fluids, and when I called the doctor, he advised me to eat soup. My blood pressure was too low and, as a result, your heart beats faster to get your blood pressure up, but it was not working.

I was so very excited. I could never eat soup while on dialysis because it had too much sodium. Now, I was told I could eat soup. I reached for chicken-flavored ramen noodles and was in heaven! The soup did help bring up my blood pressure, which then decreased my heart rate, but I was still having episodes of the low blood pressure and high heart rates, especially in the morning and evening. Finally, I couldn't take it anymore. I called the transplant surgeon on call, and he said to get to the Emergency Room immediately. He suggested the University of Michigan Health System would be best since I just had a transplant there. We got to the Emergency Room around 11 p.m., and I was treated with lots of fluids. It is very hard to drink two liters of liquid a day when you are used to holding back. It took me months to get on the right track.

I was eventually put on unit 5C around noon the next day and was in the hospital until Saturday when my dad and husband picked me up.

They had been creating a bromance while I was away in the hospital! I think they both enjoyed getting to know each other better. The doctors decided they needed to adjust my blood pressure medicine and felt it would be better to do this through the clinic instead of keeping me in the hospital. Keep in mind, beds on 5C are hot commodities! After returning home, I went to the clinic weekly for about two months and then they spread out my visits to every two weeks for one month, then every three weeks.

My recovery took much longer than my previous transplant. Fourteen years before, I had been back to work in five weeks. This time, at five weeks I still felt horrible and was in lots of pain. I was not moving around much, and I was sleeping a lot. I was not healing as well since I was inactive. The problem was that when I would start moving around, my heart rate would increase and I would start feeling bad.

I went back to work after two months and decided to start slowly. I started with 20 hours the first week, 30 hours the second week, and 40 hours the third week. By the sixth week, I finally started to feel like myself again. I was tired, but no longer in constant pain at my transplant site. Since then, I have started doing more things and walking more and farther.

My three-month biopsy came out great! No rejection and no donor-specified antibodies. This was wonderful news, especially since this was my third transplant. I was feeling so blessed!

I started not feeling well at the end of June 2017 but could not attribute it to any kidney issue. I thought I had a sinus infection or a touch of a bug, but I had no fever. After being out of work a couple of days, I went to the local Emergency Room to make sure my heart was okay. I had a urinary tract infection (UTI) and was given a prescription for antibiotics and sent home. They checked my labs and the kidney was good. I was unable to get the antibiotics until three days later. I do not recommend this since the infection can get to your kidney very quickly. I had never done this before in 25 years.

Thursday, July 6, I had my regular labs drawn and my creatinine had tripled from 1.16 to 3.35. I was told to go straight to the Emergency Room. I had a blockage between my transplanted ureter and bladder, which was causing fluid to collect in my kidney, and that was causing my creatinine to go up. I was admitted and had a tube put into my kidney to drain the urine until the obstruction could be corrected. I will use a nephrostomy bag until I get an appointment with the urologist to either put a stent between the ureter and bladder or to have surgery to move the ureter to another location on the bladder. I had my original, postsurgical stent removed three weeks early because it was causing so much irritation. This may be one of the reasons for the obstruction, along with not treating the UTI immediately.

I will take each day as it comes and try to be positive. Today is my first day back to work with the nephrostomy bag; I'm using leg straps to keep the bag attached to my leg while wearing stretch jeans. It is a perfect combination.

As I learn each day, it is a journey, and I never know what is going to happen from day to day. Of all the things to know about kidney transplants, these are the ones that stand out:

- Always be your own best advocate. Pay attention to your medications and follow doctor's orders. You know your body the best. Make sure you can explain how you are feeling, as this will help the doctors to correct your issue.

- Leave your dignity at home. I lost it when I was young, and I don't even think about it anymore. Doctors will end up seeing everything as we age, anyway.
- Pack a lot of patience. Being in the hospital is not a quick process. If they tell you that you will be released soon, that means three or four hours. Just stay relaxed and watch television, read a book, or take a nap. I don't even change my clothes until they bring the release papers.
- Keep a positive attitude! My philosophy is, "Keep smiling and people will wonder what you are up to." A positive attitude makes all the difference in the world. You will be a pleasant patient and doctors will be more likely to listen to you and help you.
- Finally, have faith! It has helped me deal with all the challenges that came my way with this process.

# Resources

### Gift of Life Michigan (GOLM)

GOLM is Michigan's organ procurement organization, dedicated to organ and tissue recovery. The organization maintains the Michigan Organ Donor Registry in partnership with the Michigan Secretary of State.

www.giftoflifemichigan.org
www.giftoflifemichigan.org/go/umhs
3861 Research Park Dr.
Ann Arbor, MI 48108
866-500-5801

### Detroit Minority Organ Tissue Transplant Education Program (Detroit MOTTEP)

This is a section of GOLM that focuses on minority organ and tissue education in the Detroit area. Detroit MOTTEP's goal is to encourage minorities to register as organ donors and to become educated about transplantation.

www.detroitmottepfoundation.org
736 Lothrop St.
Detroit, MI 48202
313-875-9055

### National Kidney Foundation of Michigan (NKFM)

NKFM is dedicated to preventing kidney disease and improving the quality of life for those who have kidney disease.

www.nkfm.org
1169 Oak Valley Dr.
Ann Arbor, MI 48108
800-482-1455

**National Living Donor Assistance Center (NLDAC)**

NLDAC provides financial assistance for organ donors. Although transplant-related medical costs are not charged to donors, NLDAC can help with the cost of travel and other expenses.
www.livingdonorassistance.org
2461 S. Clark St.
Suite 640
Arlington, VA 22202
888-870-5002

**United Network of Organ Sharing (UNOS)**

UNOS is the organization that oversees the country's organ procurement policies and procedures. UNOS strives to improve organ availability and transplantation on a national level.
www.unos.org
700 N. 4th St.
Richmond, VA 23219
804-782-4800

**University of Michigan Transplant Center**

The University of Michigan Transplant Center is a part of Michigan Medicine dedicated to saving lives through organ transplantation. Since 1964, more than 6,600 kidney transplants have taken place through the U-M Transplant Center, where Michigan Medicine continues to pursue the latest technologies and methods the field has to offer.
www.uofmhealth.org/transplant
1500 E. Medical Center Dr.
Taubman Center Fl. 1 Rec. G
Ann Arbor, MI 48109
800-333-9013

**University of Michigan Transplant Center Peer Mentors**

At the University of Michigan Transplant Center patients and family members have the opportunity to speak with an individual who has received or donated a kidney. Prospective donors and recipients can hear about their experiences and ask questions as they move through their transplant journey.

www.uofmhealth.org/transplant
300 N. Ingalls St.
Room 5D17
Ann Arbor, MI 48109
transplantoutreach@umich.edu
800-333-9013

**Wolverines for Life**

A partnership between the University of Michigan, Gift of Life Michigan, Eversight, Be the Match, and the American Red Cross, with a mission of advocating for organ, tissue, bone marrow, and blood donation. The partnership hosts donor drives throughout the University of Michigan campus and beyond in an effort to decrease organ, blood, and bone marrow waitlist deaths.

www.wolverinesforlife.org
300 N. Ingalls St.
Room 5D17
Ann Arbor, MI 48109
734-998-0095

**U.S. Department of Health & Human Services (Division of Transplantation)**

Official federal site for the Division of Transplantation. DoT is responsible for increasing organ donor registration and donation.

www.organdonor.gov

# About the Editor

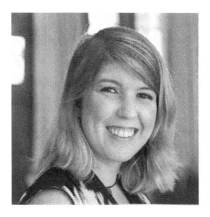

Megan Podschlne is the Project Manager at the University of Michigan Transplant Center. She began working as the Center's Outreach Assistant in 2014 after graduating from Michigan State University with a Bachelor of Arts in Communications with a specialization in Public Relations. In 2017, she received an MBA in Management from Amberton University.

In her current position, she serves as the Program Manager of Wolverines for Life, a partnership between the University of Michigan, Gift of Life Michigan, Eversight, Be the Match, and the American Red Cross. She coordinates donor drives and leads several student organizations to advocate for life-saving donation. She also manages some of the Center's strategic planning initiatives and aids in community outreach endeavors.

*The Shapes of Memory Loss: Stories, Poems and Essays*
*from the University of Michigan Medical School and Health System*
Edited by Nan Barbas, Laura Rice-Oeschger, and Cassie Starback

**Coming Soon!**
*Chronic Obstructive Pulmonary Disease: A Collection of Personal Stories*
Edited by Sara K. Whisenant and Mary Kay Hamby

*Your Transplant Adventure: A Kid's Guide to Organ Transplant*
Written by Matt Butler, LMSW, and Tanya Smith, LMSW

You can find these titles on Amazon.

35070801R00093

Made in the USA
Middletown, DE
04 February 2019